SOCIAL COMPETENCE, SYMPTOMS AND UNDERACHIEVEMENT IN CHILDHOOD:

A Longitudinal Perspective

SOCIAL COMPETENCE, SYMPTOMS AND UNDERACHIEVEMENT IN CHILDHOOD:

A Longitudinal Perspective

MARTIN KOHN

1977

V. H. WINSTON & SONS
Washington, D.C.

A HALSTED PRESS BOOK

JOHN WILEY & SONS
New York   Toronto   London   Sydney

V. H. Winston & Sons, a Division of Scripta Technica, Inc.,
Publishers
1511 K St. N. W., Washington, D. C. 20005

Distributed solely by Halsted Press, a Division of John Wiley
& Sons, Inc.

Library of Congress Cataloging in Publication Data

Kohn, Martin.
  Social competence, symptoms and underachievement in
childhood.

  Bibliography: p.
  Includes indexes.
  1. Child psychology—Longitudinal studies. 2. Child
mental health. 3. Mentally ill children. 4. Underachievers.
I. Title.
BF721.K64   155.4'18   77-5011
ISBN 0-470-99151-8

Composition by **Marie A. Maddalena**, Scripta Technica, Inc.

Contents

v

List of Tables

List of Figures

Acknowledgements

I would like to acknowledge my indebtedness to some of the many individuals and organizations without whose assistance the present study could not have been carried out.

I am particularly indebted to the Division of Day Care of the New York City Department of Social Services and its Director, Miss Muriel Katz, and Chief Educational Consultant, Miss Florence Kennedy, without whose interest and active support the study could not have been undertaken; to the directors of the 90 day care centers who cooperated wholeheartedly in the study; and to the Day Care Council of New York, particularly Mrs. Marjorie Grosett, for facilitating our work in the day care centers.

I am also indebted to the Board of Education of the City of New York, and especially to Mrs. Betty Winton, Director of the Division of Early Education, without whose help the longitudinal follow-up of the children could not have taken place. After day care many of the children went to parochial schools, and I am indebted to Mrs. Frederick Thompson, who was, until her retirement, Consultant for School Health to the Office of the Superintendent of Schools of the Archdiocese of New York, and to the Reverend Vincent D. Breen, Superintendent of Schools of the Diocese of Brooklyn, for their able assistance in the longitudinal follow-up of the parochial school pupils. Needless to say, I am indebted to the hundreds of day care and elementary school teachers who so consistently and conscientiously provided the data for the study.

ix

I am deeply indebted to all the members of my staff whose diligent work made this effort possible. I want to single out particularly Dr. Helen Silverman who assumed major responsibility for developing the preschool instruments; Dr. Jane Knitzer who obtained the initial random sample of 1,232 children; Mrs. Barbara Parnes who monitored the longitudinal follow-up and supervised the data analysis; and Dr. Bernice Rosman who ably helped me to coordinate all phases of the work and collaborated on the preparation of several journal articles. I also want to thank the numerous students, enrolled in work-study programs at Antioch College, Beloit College, and Goddard College, who helped with data collection and preparation of the data for computer analysis.

I am deeply thankful to Dr. Earl S. Schaefer for permission to use his Classroom Behavior Inventory and for the generous advice and encouragement he provided throughout.

I am indebted to Dr. Jacob Cohen who, as statistical consultant, guided me in the application of multivariate analytic procedures and whose helpful counsel was graciously given many times.

This study was funded in part by National Institute of Mental Health grants #13588 and #16944. I am particularly grateful to Dr. A. Hussain Tuma whose valuable support and guidance greatly encouraged our efforts. I am also indebted to the William Alanson White Institute, especially its Director, Dr. Earl G. Witenberg, and Mr. Mel Gordon, President, for providing an atmosphere conducive to research and for generosity in underwriting the final stages of the project.

Finally, but certainly not least, I am indebted to my wife, Vera, for her devoted help in editing the manuscript. Her patience and support made it possible for me to bring this project to completion.

M. K.

Introductory Commentary

In this volume, Martin Kohn has provided a confluence of two important streams of contemporary psychological research. One, the study of *competence* has, until recent years, been the victim of benign neglect by both researchers *and* clinicians interested in developmental processes in children; the other, *symptom formation* (or the signs of deviant personality functioning, if you will) has long been the province of those involved in diagnosing and treating disturbed children and adults. A word about each in turn.

The relative neglect by developmental psychologists of the origins and attributes of competent behavior, other than intellectual functioning, is one of those strange paradoxes in our scientific life to which Lois Murphy has earlier given voice. I have quoted the following passage from *The Widening World of Childhood* so frequently as to warrant the payment of royalties to Dr. Murphy and her colleagues, but allow me one more go at it.

At the very beginning of that volume, which bears the significant subtitle, *Paths Toward Mastery*, Dr. Murphy (1962) writes as follows:

"It is something of a paradox that a nation which has exulted in its rapid expansion and its scientific-technological achievements, should have developed in its studies of childhood so vast a "problem" literature: a literature often expressing adjustment difficulties, social failures, blocked potentialities, and defeat. Since it came parallel with the muckraking and social criticism literature of the first half of the twentieth century, its emergence may, indeed, be considered partly due to different phases in our American history. Pioneer courage and the will to do were crystallized in the mottoes of the nineteenth century; in the twentieth century we became preoccupied with failures. In applying clinical ways of thinking formulated out of experience with broken adults, we were slow to see how the language of adequacy to meet life's challenges could become the subject matter of psychological science. Thus there are thousands of studies of maladjustment for each one that deals directly with the ways of managing life's problems with personal strength and adequacy. The language of problems, difficulties, inadequacies, of antisocial or delinquent conduct, or of ambivalence and anxiety is familiar. We know that there are devices for correcting, bypassing, or overcoming threats, but for the most part these have not been directly studied" (p. 2).

Fortunately, since Murphy first wrote these words in 1962, a change has slowly been generated by child psychologists. The revitalization of developmental psychology over the past two decades, both in terms of methodology and theory, has begun to provide a new and more complex set of contents that can help better to explain the development of healthy as well as deviant personality formation in children. Studies of the redemptive power of early peer play, the significance of modeling and reinforcement in initiating and sustaining behavior, the nature of attachment and its evidential role in patterning separation and stranger anxiety, the impact of longitudinal and cross-sectional research in assessing cognitive and affective growth and the development of socialization have begun to provide the foundation stones for a developmental psychopathology markedly different from the child psychiatry and the child clinical psychology that exists today.

Lest I add too optimistic a note regarding the current climate of research on competence, I must note that despite the appearance of significant volumes such as those by Coelho, Hamburg, and Adams (1974), Murphy and Moriarty (1976), Connolly and Bruner (1974), and White and Watt (1973) that help to document the adaptive quality of individuals under neutral or stressful naturalistic conditions, we remain relatively neglectful in studying the emergence of competence in children and adults.

Shortly before these comments were written, our Minnesota research group had decided to attempt a definitive review of the present status of research on the nature of competence in normal and deviant children. Our small group delved into the *Psychological Abstracts* and quickly affirmed that competence is not an ascriptor term in the indices and that an adequate canvass of the literature could only be assured were we to cover a wide range of ascriptors of which these are merely representative: *achievement, adaptation, social adjustment, personality adjustment, pre-school* and *school age children, coping, emotional security, emotional maturity, emotional stability, mental health, psychological stress, psychosocial development, self-esteem, stress reaction,* etc. Obviously the generic quality of competence remains sufficiently unrecognized by abstracters that it cannot yet compete with the traditionalism of these alternative terms.

Dr. Kohn's second interest lies in the area of *symptom formation* and here we are on more familiar grounds. The literature of behavior pathology is vast and embedded within that literature are research studies that attest to the profound importance of competence as a variable significantly implicated both in resistance to the encroachment of psychopathology or to rapidity of recovery (i.e., favorable prognosis) when breakdown occurs. Here is a relatively stable literature in an area of notorious instability. Phillips (1953, 1968), in collaboration with his colleague Zigler (Zigler & Phillips, 1960, 1961), produced a series of important studies at the Worcester State Hospital demonstrating that premorbid competence, as indexed by such factors as occupational level, education, job stability, peer relationships in childhood and adulthood, and intellectual performance, related powerfully both to the form of psychopathology manifested during disorder and to recovery from disorder if it occurred. Their observation that symptoms marked by "turning against the self" tended to be correlated with indicators of good premorbid competence, whereas those marked by "turning against others" or "withdrawal from others" were accompanied by behavior that reflected premorbid incompetence added power to a prognostic literature that emphasizes two constellations in schizophrenic disorders: reactive schizophrenia/premorbid competence/recovery vs. process schizophrenia/premorbid incompetence/relapse

(Garmezy, 1970a; Kantor & Herron, 1966; Zigler & Phillips, 1962; Zubin, Sutton, Salzinger, Salzinger, Burdock, & Peretz, 1961).

In the continuing controversy over continuity or discontinuity in life span developmental psychology, two of the most severe forms of psychopathology, chronic schizophrenia and antisocial personality disorder ("withdrawal from others" and "turning against others"), appear to lean heavily in the direction of the continuity of incompetence from childhood or (more typically) adolescence through adulthood.

Nevertheless, I wish to avoid stating this element of continuity in terms of formal nosology, cognizant of Michael Rutter's (1972) review that some behavior disorders seem to reflect a relationship between child and adult psychiatric disorders while others do not. Classified more clearly within the first category would be "psychopathy"; adult "psychopaths" are more likely than not to have shown repeated antisocial acts in childhood, whereas only half the children with earlier acting-out patterns will continue such behaviors in adulthood. By contrast, however, schizophrenia would have to be assigned to the second category as would childhood neuroses (which often prove to be quite transitory and unrepresented in adulthood if the earlier behaviors reflect exaggerations of normal developmental trends) and childhood depression and adult depression which fail to show clearly established lines of continuity.

I will return to the problem of testing continuity or discontinuity hypotheses shortly. But before doing so, it is necessary to provide a brief citation of one aspect of symptom formation that does suggest a similarity between childhood and adult psychopathology. The clusters of adult behaviors identified as "turning against the self" vs. "turning against others" finds a parallel in what Kohn prefers to call "the two-factor model of social-emotional functioning." This model identifies two major syndromes that appear and reappear in the literature of childhood psychopathology. Hewitt and Jenkins (1946) identified behavioral clusters that they termed "overinhibited," "unsocialized aggressive," and "socialized delinquent" children. Jenkins (1964) subsequently referred to "inhibited" vs. "aggressive" groups of disturbed children. Peterson (1961) and others described a "personality problem" vs. "conduct problem" dichotomy, and Bennett (1960) in a British study compared "neurotic" and "delinquent" children. At Minnesota, Achenbach's (1966) factor-analytic study of 300 male and 300 female psychiatric patients (ages 4-15) who had been seen in a child psychiatric unit of a University hospital produced a first principal bipolar factor with antisocial (i.e., "externalizing") behavior at one end and symptoms of "internalizing" behavior at the other. A recent study by the Minnesota group of a large number of children seen in a community child guidance clinic reaffirms the presence of these factors, but seemingly as unipolar dimensions. Dr. Kohn's second chapter provides a review of this important aspect of childhood psychopathology.

In a review (Garmezy, 1970b) of the correlates of this behavioral dichotomy in disturbed children it has been shown that factors present in both child and parent differentiated the externalizing children from their internalizing counterparts: Reduced competence served as a marker for the acting-out group while higher competence attributes were more characteristic of the neurotic children. Furthermore, follow-up studies by Robins (1966), Shea (1972), and others strongly suggest a pattern of reduced competence and more manifest pathology in adulthood evidenced by antisocial children in comparison with their more inhibited, neurotic controls.

Thus, a restricted convergence appears to be evident between competence in childhood and adulthood and highly specific forms of early and later symptom formation. Nevertheless, the scaffolding for such a hierarchical developmental structure is rather weak. Divergent cross-sectional groups mark the reviews of childhood vs. adult psychopathology. Furthermore, the number of cases in these studies tends to be small, procedures are often non-comparable, and criteria for adaptation frequently poorly defined. As for follow-up studies, these are few and far between in childhood disorders and when present, suffer the attrition that is commonplace in longitudinal research—an attrition that is even more accentuated in a deviant population.

Where does the ultimate solution to this critical problem of both outcome and continuity in psychopathology lie? It probably is to be found in a national large-scale, collaborative, longitudinal study of children at risk for present and future behavior disorder. But this likelihood is not part of a realistic present and may even be exempt from an unknown future. However, one can conceive of an intermediate step that would involve the support of a series of relatively short-term longitudinal studies over the developmental span from the preschool years to middle childhood to adolescence, from adolescence to early maturity, and finally from early adulthood to the middle years of life.

A most trying venture, but one must start somewhere, and this brings us to Martin Kohn's *Social Competence, Symptoms and Underachievement in Childhood: A Longitudinal Perspective*, a title that provides the author's own summary of his impressive pioneering effort.

Longitudinal studies not only generate subject attrition, but they erode investigators as well. It is, therefore, all the more of a tribute to the author that he set out to examine the "longitudinal persistence of emotional impairment for a five-year period." His span of investigation embraced his subjects' preschool years to their attendance in the fourth grade of New York City's elementary schools.

Of 92 public day care centers in the city that came under the jurisdiction of the Division of Day Care of the city's Department of Social Services, only two declined to participate. Taking a random 20% sample from these day care centers, the author began this major longitudinal effort with 1,232 children who ranged in age from 3-6 years and were divided almost equally between boys and girls. A social class distribution ranging from lower to middle class was represented with both minority and white youngsters present in sufficiently large numbers as to enable the author to derive conclusions that possess a reasonable degree of stability. Data on the children were collected at regular intervals over the five-year period—a fact that improves on the typical follow-up study and provides the base for what has been termed a "follow-through" investigation.

The rate of attrition is a tribute to the author's dedication: A 74%-79% return during the fifth year of data collection represents an excellent follow-up count, given current patterns of urban mobility. Unfortunately, attrition tended to be somewhat more selective, with a larger proportion of deviant children who were lost to the study. Such a finding comes as no surprise to any psychopathologist who lives with this as a major fact of his or her research life. But enough children remained to warrant serious attention to this research project.

Like with any good story, the writer of a preface should not reveal the ending. But I cannot restrain offering some observations about this study. I offer these:

1. This study does not set deviant apart from healthy adaptation. The instruments devised and used by the author provide polarities marked by positive attributes at one end, disturbing ones at the other;

2. The critical importance of identifying *potentially* disturbed preschool children provides the base for early intervention efforts. This volume is a way station toward the recognition of those early signs of inadequate functioning that can help to generate positive efforts at primary prevention. On the positive side, too, the ready identification of healthy children in underprivileged settings is of equal importance to the well-being of family, community, and nation;

3. Emotional impairment and academic underachievement go hand in hand. These are the unwelcome progenitors of an ecological model (Birch & Gussow, 1970) for the transgenerational relationship between poverty and educational failure that too often is the lot of our socially disadvantaged citizens.

The many additional findings of this significant study I leave to the reader.

A comment about the author: Martin Kohn represents that interesting combination of education and background that often marks the sophisticated psychopathologist. Trained in two departments marked by a rigorous adherence to the experimental tradition in psychology—the Johns Hopkins University and Yale University (where he was a research assistant to Professor Neal E. Miller)—his interests subsequently turned to the study of children as evidenced by the research positions he has held with the Jewish Board of Guardians, the Bank Street College of Education, the William Alanson White Institute, the New York State Division of Youth, and the Board of Education of the City of New York.

Thirteen years of NIMH grant support to the William Alanson White Institute, for which Dr. Kohn has served as Principal Investigator, have been devoted to the development of screening procedures for emotionally disturbed preschool children, the individualization of training of these children to enhance their classroom competence, followed by the creation of instruments necessary to assess major dimensions of social competence and symptom patterning in the children—all culminating in the longitudinal study that is described in this volume.

Here, then, is the product of a seasoned investigator trained in psychology's experimental traditions as well as its clinical applications.

This volume has had a lengthy incubation. It deserves attention.

Norman Garmezy

Minneapolis, Minnesota
January, 1977

REFERENCES

Achenbach, T. M. The classification of children's psychiatric symptoms: A factor analytic study. *Psychological Monographs*, 1966, **80**, #6, No. 615, 37 pp.

Bennett, I. *Delinquent and neurotic children*. New York: Basic Books, 1960.

Birch, H. G., & Gussow, J. D. *Disadvantaged children: Health, nutrition and social failure*. New York: Harcourt, Brace & World, 1970.

Coelho, G. V., Hamburg, D. A., & Adams, J. E. (Eds.), *Coping and adaptation*. New York: Basic Books, 1974.

Connolly, K. J., & Bruner, J. S. (Eds.), *The growth of competence*. New York: Academic Press, 1974.

Garmezy, N. Process and reactive schizophrenia: Some conceptions and issues. *Schizophrenia Bulletin*, 1970, **2**, 30—74. (a)

Garmezy, N. Vulnerable children: Implications derived from studies of an internalizing-externalizing symptom dimension.

In J. Zubin & A. M. Freedman (Eds.), *The psychopathology of adolescence.* New York: Grune & Stratton, 1970, pp. 212–239. (b)

Hewitt, L. E., & Jenkins, R. L. *Fundamental patterns of maladjustment: The dynamics of their origin.* Springfield, Illinois: D. H. Green, 1946.

Jenkins, R. L. Diagnoses, dynamics, and treatment in child psychiatry. In R. L. Jenkins & J. O. Cole (Eds.), Diagnostic classification in child psychiatry. Washington, D.C. *Psychiatric Research Reports of the American Psychiatric Association,* 1964, **18,** 91–120.

Kantor, R. E., & Herron, W. G. *Reactive and process schizophrenia,* Palo Alto, Calif.: Science & Behavior Books, 1966.

Murphy, L., & collaborators. *The widening world of childhood.* New York: Basic Books, 1962.

Murphy, L. B., & Moriarty, A. E. *Vulnerability, coping and growth.* New Haven: Yale University Press, 1976.

Peterson, D. R. Behavior problems of middle childhood. *Journal of Consulting Psychology,* 1961, **25,** 205–209.

Phillips, L. Case history data & prognosis in schizophrenia. *Journal of Nervous & Mental Disease,* 1953, **6,** 515–525.

Phillips, L. *Human adaptation and its failures.* New York: Academic Press, 1968.

Robins, L. N. *Deviant children grown up.* Baltimore, Md.: Williams & Wilkins, 1966.

Rutter, M. L. Relationships between child and adult psychiatric disorders: Some research considerations. *Acta Psychiatrica Scandinavica,* 1972, **48,** 3–21.

Shea, M. J. *A follow-up study into adulthood of adolescent psychiatric patients in relation to internalizing and externalizing symptoms, MMPI configurations, social competence and life history variables.* Unpublished doctoral dissertation, University of Minnesota, 1972.

White, B. L., & Watts, J. C. *Experience and environment.* Englewood Cliffs, N.J.: Prentice-Hall, 1973.

Zigler, E., & Phillips, L. Social effectiveness and symptomatic behaviors. *Journal of Abnormal and Social Psychology,* 1960, **61,** 231–238.

Zigler, E., & Phillips, L. Social competence and outcome in psychiatric disorder. *Journal of Abnormal and Social Psychology*, 1961, **63**, 264–271.

Zigler, E., & Phillips, L. Social competence and the process-reactive distinction in psychopathology. *Journal of Abnormal and Social Psychology*, 1962, **65**, 215–222.

Zubin, J., Sutton, S., Salzinger, K., Salzinger, S., Burdock, E. I., & Peretz, D. A biometric approach to prognosis in schizophrenia. In P. H. Hoch & J. Zubin (Eds.), *Comparative epidemiology of the mental disorders*. New York: Grune & Stratton, 1961, pp. 143–203.

CHAPTER 1
Author's Introduction

The present study was an outgrowth of a previous research project designed to determine the effectiveness of a program of therapeutic intervention with emotionally disturbed children in day care (Kohn & Rosman, 1971).

The earlier project was carried out in six New York day care centers with a total population of slightly over 400 children. In order to select the most disturbed of these 400 children as well as to determine the nature of their disturbance, two teacher rating instruments—the Symptom Checklist and the Social Competence Scale—were developed. The Symptom Checklist was designed to assess the presence or absence of behavior generally considered symptomatic of disturbance in the preschool child; the Social Competence Scale was designed to assess the child's mastery of the preschool environment. Every child was rated on both instruments independently by the two full-time teachers in the classroom.

In order to reduce the massive amount of information generated by the two instruments to manageable proportions and at the same time to determine the major dimensions of symptoms and social competence, each instrument was subjected to a factor analysis. The Symptom Checklist yielded two major factors which were called:

Factor I: Apathy-Withdrawal
Factor II: Anger-Defiance

The Social Competence Scale also yielded two major factors; these were bipolar and were labeled:

Factor I: Interest-Participation versus Apathy-Withdrawal
Factor II: Cooperation-Compliance versus Anger-Defiance

Correlational analysis showed that the two major factor dimensions of the Symptom Checklist and the two major dimensions of the Social Competence Scale measured the same behavior patterns; that is to say, the child who scored high on Apathy-Withdrawal on one instrument tended to score high on Apathy-Withdrawal on the other, and similarly for Anger-Defiance. The principal difference between the two instruments was that the Symptom Checklist measured varying degrees of pathology whereas the Social Competence Scale measured the whole range of functioning from health to disturbance and, therefore, permitted discrimination not only of varying degrees of disturbance but also of varying degrees of healthy functioning.

The emergence of these two syndromes provided the major impetus for the work reported in this book. The two dimensions had frequently appeared during the last 50 years in the work of other researchers studying emotional disturbance in children, and the recurrence of the findings seemed to me to have potentially great theoretical as well as practical significance. To date this potential had not been realized because:

1. Each team of investigators had generally invented their

own designations for the syndromes which emerged from their particular study; this had led to a confusing proliferation of labels and obscured the fact that similar dimensions of functioning were being found in studies encompassing a wide variety of subjects, age groups, settings, and instruments.

2. Investigators who observed that, in spite of the differences in terminology, the same basic syndromes were being identified confined their analyses to "armchair" approaches: They either pointed to the semantic similarity of the items which went into the two recurring symptom clusters (see Eysenck, 1970), or they related the various study results to each other by demonstrating their place in a circumplex model of social-emotional functioning (see Emmerich, 1977; Schaefer, 1961, 1971).

The objective of the present study was to take a bold step forward and demonstrate the usefulness of the two-factor model in a longitudinal study which had three major foci of interest:

1. The epidemiology of emotional impairment and academic underachievement in childhood;
2. The longitudinal persistence of emotional impairment;
3. The relationship between emotional impairment and academic underachievement.

Before we could undertake the study, two basic issues had to be settled. First, it was important to demonstrate empirically that the two syndromes which had emerged from representative studies were in fact the same or at least very similar patterns of behavior regardless of what the investigators had labeled them. The only way to secure empirical evidence was to apply measuring instruments developed for different studies to the same subjects and to obtain correlation coefficients among dimensions hypothesized to be congruent. The larger the correlations, the more definite the conclusion that the instruments measured the same phenomena and that the different labels referred to the same behavior patterns.

Second, it was necessary to demonstrate that the two dimensions had clinical relevance. Many of the earlier studies were based on clinical samples, i.e., children who had been referred for treatment because of emotional disturbance or who had been diagnosed as emotionally impaired. With clinical samples the two syndromes seem to make a valid differentiation in terms of the types of behavior patterns that children manifest and the kind of symptomatology they display. In the present study the subjects were to be a randomly selected group of "normal" children, some of whom were healthier than others. Consequently, we had to ascertain whether the factor dimensions of the Symptom Checklist and the Social Competence Scale were in fact related to the health-disturbance continuum, i.e., whether they would differentiate the more disturbed from the less disturbed and identify those children who were in need of psychiatric or psychological attention.

Once these issues were resolved, we could address ourselves to the principal purpose of the study.

Epidemiology of Emotional Impairment and Academic Underachievement

Two of the major psychological handicaps afflicting children are emotional impairment and academic underachievement. The incidence of both disorders is high (see Clancy & Smither, 1953; Coleman, 1966; Gilbert, 1957; Lurie, 1970; Rogers, 1942; Ullman, 1952).

Emotional impairment

The wide prevalence of emotional disorders, the length and costliness of individual treatment as well as hope that prevention or intervention programs could be formulated on a community-wide basis have in recent decades stimulated researchers to adopt an epidemiological approach and look to the social milieu for the causes and roots of emotional disturbance. Evidence accumulated which made it plausible to assume that, as Srole, Langner, Michael, Opler, and Rennie (1962) put it: "Socio-cultural conditions, in both their normative and deviant forms, operating in intrafamily and extrafamily settings during childhood and adulthood have measurable consequences reflected in the mental health differences to be observed within a population" (p. 13).

As Dohrenwend and Dohrenwend (1969) have shown in their review of epidemiological studies of psychiatric disorders, there is considerable evidence that among adults (age 20 and over) prevalence of emotional impairment varies inversely with social status. Some observers hold that the lower-class adult's more difficult and stressful life situation leads to emotional disturbance; others believe that the lower-class youngster enters adulthood with a heavy burden of psychological damage acquired in childhood (see also Michael, 1962). However, investigations involving children have yielded conflicting evidence on the extent to which the sociocultural matrix in which the child is embedded has a decisive influence on his emotional well-being.

In the present study the relationship between emotional impairment and social class and minority-group membership was of particular interest. A major objective was to determine (a) whether children's emotional impairment was a function of their parents' social-class and minority-group status, and (b) whether evidence for the existence of the relationship could be found in the early and middle years of childhood, i.e., between the ages of 3 and 10. Positive findings would then demand further research to ascertain whether the causal factors were social or constitutional/genetic. If no evidence was found, much of what has been said about the deleterious effect of lower-class life on social-emotional functioning would need to be reconsidered.

In addition to examining the impact of variables covering the sociocultural environment in which the children were growing up, it was planned to study emotional impairment as a function of sex and age.

Academic underachievement

Academic attainment was to be similarly related to age, sex, and background factors relevant to the sociocultural matrix in which the child was embedded. In contrast to emotional impairment on which the rescarch evidence is limited, a great deal is known about the relationship between academic impairment and lower-class and minority-group status. The poor scholastic record of "disadvantaged" children has been ascribed to genetic (Jensen, 1968), constitutional (Pasamanick & Knobloch, 1961), and environmental (Bernstein, 1961; Dave, 1963; Deutsch & Associates, 1967; McClelland, 1961; Moles, 1965; Wolf, 1963) factors. Whatever the cause or causes, the link between academic performance and sociocultural background is well-established.

In the present study we focused on the question of whether, as has been widely assumed in recent years (see, e.g., Irelan, 1966; Joint Commission on Mental Health of Children, 1969; Moles, 1965), the variables relevant to the advantaged-disadvantaged continuum would show the same relationship to the achievement criteria as to the measures of social-emotional functioning.

Longitudinal Persistence of Emotional Impairment

The longitudinal persistence of emotional impairment is one of the unanswered questions in childhood psychopathology. Some psychoanalysts and students of personality development believe that emotional disturbance in childhood is always a handicap to healthy development. Others, like Anna Freud (1946/1965), disagree: "This impression of a serious hold-up is frequently misleading. After a shorter or a longer stay, symptoms may suddenly lose importance; the fixation can dissolve and the libido, freed from restrictions, resume its normal progressive flow. The child has, as the popular saying goes, 'outgrown' its neurosis, and therapeutic help has become unnecessary," (pp. 80–81). Similar views have been expressed by Shepherd, Oppenheim, and Mitchell (1971) and White (1952).

The evidence from systematic research efforts is not conclusive but tends to suggest a trend in the direction of persistence. For example, working with a "normal" sample, Macfarlane, Allen, and Honzik (1954) found moderate-to-strong persistence in total number of problems for two phases of development: (a) from preschool (ages 3 to 5) to preadolescence (ages 9 to 11)—no persistence beyond that age level; and (b) from early school period (age 6) to adolescence (ages 12 to 14).

The data of Robins (1966) indicated that a high proportion of preadolescents and adolescents referred for treatment to a child guidance clinic showed symptoms of serious pathology in adulthood.

The two syndromes of emotional impairment of the present study have been found in youngsters ranging from kindergarten level to adolescence. But the fact that the same dimensions have appeared over a wide range does not necessarily imply longitudinal persistence, i.e., that a particular child will continue to manifest the same syndrome of disturbance as he grows older. Kessler (1966) has stated: "There are surveys of the prevalence of emotional disturbance—that is, both old and new cases are counted together—and they give no idea of the duration of the disturbed behavior. An indeterminate number, at any given time, have problems which will be spontaneously resolved. Unfortunately, there are few longitudinal studies of children with problems so there is no 'natural history' for emotional disorders to compare with the 'natural history' for organic illnesses" (p. 485).

Our plan was to study the longitudinal persistence of emotional impairment for a five-year period. We were primarily concerned with ascertaining whether a specific syndrome would remain stable over time, i.e.: (a) whether children who manifested a particular type of disturbance (e.g., Apathy-Withdrawal or Anger-Defiance on the Symptom Checklist and Social Competence Scale) would show the same syndrome a few years later, and (b) whether children who displayed a particular pattern of health (Interest-Participation or Cooperation-Compliance on the Social Competence Scale) would exhibit the same pattern of health a few years later. If evidence of persistence was found, the way would be opened for early identification of children at risk and investigation into those factors in the child's make-up or in his family and social situation which cause and perpetuate pathology. Positive results would permit early detection of youngsters showing healthy functioning and research as to possible biological or social determinants of emotional well-being. If the data pointed to behavioral change rather than stability, research would be needed to investigate factors which lead to remission of symptoms or cause a healthy child to become disturbed.

The findings would also have implications for programs of therapeutic intervention since, as was shown in Kohn and Rosman (1971), a different treatment approach is needed for each syndrome of emotional impairment.

Relationship between Emotional Impairment and Academic Underachievement

Emotional impairment and academic underachievement have frequently been found to be related to each other, both in clinical studies (see Katan, 1961; Pearson, 1952) and in systematic research investigations (see Bower, 1969; Harris, 1961; Olson, 1930; Stennett, 1966). To date, research findings have been somewhat ambiguous, however, for two reasons:

1. Research and hypothesis formulation have been hampered because emotional disturbance has been conceptualized along one of two extremes: Either emotional impairment has been seen as a single continuum, ranging from healthy to disturbed; or theorizing has been so refined (e.g., Freud took the position that no symptom was fully understood unless genetic, structural, and psychodynamic factors were taken into account) that no present methodology can expect to cope fully with these complex formulations.

2. Most of the research studies have been carried out with school-age children. For this age group no clear-cut conclusions can be drawn about the direction of cause and effect: After the child has entered school, his emotional impairment may lead to underachievement; however, the converse may also be true, and failure to achieve may lead to emotional impairment.

About a decade ago Bateman (1966) pointed out that in spite of the importance of the topic both to child development and clinical theory, few systematic studies have used preschool social-emotional functioning as the predictor variable and intellectual achievement as the dependent variable. Except for the work in this laboratory (Kohn & Rosman, 1972a, 1973a), nothing has been published in the years since the appearance of Bateman's review to contradict her conclusion.

In the present study data on the Symptom Checklist and the Social Competence Scale were to be gathered prior to the onset of formal education and related to the children's subsequent school performance. We were particularly interested in determining (a) whether the child who was emotionally disturbed during the preschool period was likely to be at risk of underachievement in elementary school, and (b) whether one syndrome of emotional impairment was more closely related to cognition deficits and poor scholastic performance than the other: Anger-Defiance, as suggested in the report of the President's Commission on Law Enforcement and Administration of Justice (1967) and by Rutter, Tizard, and Whitmore (1970), or Apathy-Withdrawal, as indicated by two previous studies conducted by the present author (Kohn, 1968; Kohn & Rosman, 1972a, 1973a) and by the findings of Richards and McCandless (1972) and Emmerich (1977).

Innovative Research Procedures

The longitudinal study covered a span of five years: Data collection began during the preschool period and ended when the children were in fourth grade. From the methodological point of view, the present study was intended as an innovative effort designed to demonstrate the feasibility of following a very large sample (more than 1,200 children) over the five-year period with relatively simple procedures.

One of the limitations of most longitudinal research to date has been that the heavy demand on resources in terms of time, effort, and money has restricted the size of the samples that have been studied. In the present study we relied primarily on two kinds of data sources: (a) measuring instruments which enabled us to make use of the relatively untapped resource of the teacher's knowledge of the children and which were adaptable to computer processing of the information, and (b) official records.

From the therapeutic intervention study (Kohn & Rosman, 1971) it was evident that the Symptom Checklist and the Social Competence Scale could be completed on sizeable groups of preschool youngsters with a fairly small investment of teacher time. In the present study we planned to use these procedures again with the preschool group and to use comparable instruments to assess the social-emotional functioning of the same children in elementary school.

School achievement data were gathered through teacher ratings and school records and, with the cooperation of the New York City Board of Education, we obtained the children's scores on standard achievement tests which are administered routinely to all pupils attending the New York City public schools.

It goes without saying that this type of large-scale study entails some sacrifice of depth of information on the individual study subject. Nothing, however, stands in the researcher's way if he wishes to collect more comprehensive sets of data on specific subsamples of the larger group. For example, if a subgroup were identified who showed chronicity of a particular impairment, it would be possible to study these subjects further by comparing them, on measures of biological functioning or social milieu, with a group of youngsters who were equally disturbed initially but subsequently recovered. The technique of identifying subsamples enables the researcher to state from what segment of a larger and more representative sample the subgroups were drawn. This feature gives the methodology an advantage over follow-up studies of high risk children who have already come for treatment.

In the present study we identified a group of children who were at risk at one age level and remained emotionally impaired as well as a group of youngsters who were at risk at one age level and went into remission but we did not collect additional data on either group.

Overview

To recapitulate, the present study sought to expand the scope of the two-factor model of social-emotional functioning by examining these questions:

1. Are the two basic syndromes which have repeatedly emerged from research studies of emotional disturbance in children the same or at least very similar patterns of behavior

irrespective of the designations which the investigators have given to the syndromes?

2. Do these two basic dimensions, when assessing the social-emotional functioning of a group of randomly selected "normal" children, have clinical significance, i.e., do they differentiate the more disturbed from the less disturbed?

3. To what extent are type and severity of emotional impairment and academic underachievement a function of the sociocultural background of the child, particularly of the social class and the ethnic group to which he belongs?

4. To what extent do emotional impairment and healthy functioning detected in preschool children persist? Does type of impairment persist so that a child who is disturbed on one dimension in the preschool period will still be disturbed on the same dimension in later years?

5. To what extent is early emotional impairment predictive of later academic attainment? Do the two syndromes, Apathy-Withdrawal and Anger-Defiance, have the same predictive value?

In addition to the substantive issues, it was the aim of the study to show that it is feasible to track a very large sample of children with relatively simple research procedures, utilizing information that may be obtained from teachers and other public sources, in this instance, the school system.

Organization of the Book

The book has been organized in the following manner: A review of selected studies in which researchers identified two principal syndromes of emotional disturbance in children is presented in chapter 2. Chapter 3 contains a description of the development of the Symptom Checklist and the Social Competence Scale as well as a report of an empirical study which demonstrated the generality of the two-factor model, i.e., that the different labels applied by diverse investigators to the syndromes did in fact refer to the same phenomena. The design and procedures of the longitudinal study are spelled out in chapter 4. A major test of the clinical validity of the factor dimensions of the Symptom Checklist and the Social Competence Scale is reported in chapter 5.

In chapter 6 sex and age trends in social-emotional functioning and academic attainment are examined. The epidemiology and longitudinal persistence of emotional impairment are discussed in chapter 7. Additional data on persistence and early identification of children at risk appear in chapter 8. In chapter 9 the relationship between emotional impairment and underachievement is analyzed.

The final chapter contains a summary of the study and a discussion of the practical and theoretical significance of the two-factor model of social-emotional functioning as well as the value of our approach within the context of risk research. In conclusion, we propose directions which future research should take.

CHAPTER 2
The Two-Factor Model of Social-Emotional Functioning

In the course of the last 50 years, two major syndromes have repeatedly emerged from investigations into emotional disturbance in children: One is a pattern of shy, withdrawn, and inhibited behavior and the other, a pattern of antisocial, aggressive, and dominating behavior. As Rutter noted in his 1967 review of the literature on childhood psychopathology, this dichotomy has been "perhaps the most universal... of all the diagnostic distinctions made in child psychiatry" (p. 164).

Classifying symptoms into two major groupings has pragmatic value for clinicians, researchers, and teachers because it identifies children who exhibit their problems in markedly different ways. The scientific value of distinguishing between the two types of impaired functioning is enhanced if the syndrome patterns can

13

be shown (a) to be differentially related to parental behavior, and (b) to have differential long-term prognostic significance.

A brief review of major research studies is the subject of this chapter.

History and Generality of the Two-Factor Model

Intuitive and clinical approach

Among the first researchers to sort and divide problems and symptoms under two rubrics were Paynter and Blanchard (1929). Working with a clinic population of 330 children, the investigators analyzed and grouped traits under the headings, "Personality difficulty" and "Behavior difficulty." Into the former category they placed characteristics such as mental conflict, inferiority feelings, fearfulness, and day dreaming, which "primarily affect the individual and his own personal adjustment; they are the types of reactions which, carried to the extreme, are found in patients suffering from nervous and mental diseases. On the other hand, they may persist in a mild form in individuals throughout life without greatly impairing economic and social efficiency, although often a source of personal unhappiness" (p. 20).

Behavior difficulties were defined as problems which, with a few exceptions, "interfere definitely with the individual's adjustment to the regulations of organized society" (p. 21). Examples were stealing, lying, truancy, fighting, and temper tantrums. Paynter and Blanchard held that "just as personality traits hint at the possibility of a later psychopathic condition, so do certain of the behavior patterns suggest the development of delinquent trends if they become chronic habits" (p. 21).

The clinical and intuitive approach of Paynter and Blanchard was continued and extended by Ackerson (1931, 1942) in a very ambitious and comprehensive study. Ackerson analyzed 5,000 cases of children referred to the Illinois Institute for Juvenile Research. The patients ranged in age from infancy to 17 years. Using slightly different terminology, he differentiated between "Personality problems" and "Conduct problems." Ackerson explained: "Our grouping of behavior problems into personality and conduct categories does not propose to rest upon any final etiological basis, but merely follows the customary use of these terms by child workers. Insofar as criteria can be set, a personality problem is commonly thought to be a relatively intrinsic trait in an individual which in an overdeveloped or exaggerated form is associated with a diagnosis of psychosis or psychopathy or similar mental disorder. It is not ordinarily considered to be deserving of punishment or amenable to it. A conduct problem, on the other hand, in an extreme form, is usually associated with commitment to a correctional institution in the case of adults, and the spanking or other overt disciplinary measures among younger children" (1931, p. 41).

After intuitively sorting behavior problems into two categories, Ackerson summed the items in each category to obtain a "personality-total" and a "conduct-total" for each child. "The *personality-total* consists of the unweighted enumeration of all undesirable personality traits noted for each child. For example, if he is noted as *seclusive* only, his personality-total is 1; if he also *day dreams*, his total is 2; if he also has *inferiority-feelings*, his total is 3; and so on. The *conduct-total* is similarly constructed. If he *steals* only, his conduct-total is 1; if he also *truants from home*, his total is 2; if he is also *quarrelsome*, his conduct-total is 3; and so on" (1942, p. 82).

The use of composite scores was a major advance in the field since it permitted the investigator to deal with two major syndromes rather than with innumerable individual traints; it was the first step toward the more sophisticated and objective procedures of cluster analysis and factor analysis.

A further contribution of Ackerson's was that he tested the validity of the groupings by correlating each with police records. It was expected that conduct-totals would be strongly related to police records and personality-totals, weakly related. Ackerson found that 17% of the boys and 11% of the girls had a record of police arrest or juvenile court appearance for reasons of misconduct. Ackerson concluded: "The validity of the conduct-total is indicated by its bi-serial correlation of about .50 for boys and .40 for girls (when the age factor is rendered constant, or 'partialed-out') with a notation of police arrest. For personality-total, the corresponding correlations with police arrest were only about .15 and .10" (1931, p. 126).

Use of "cluster analysis"

A pioneering work in the development of a system for classifying the emotional problems of children was reported by Hewitt and Jenkins in 1946. These investigators went beyond the clinical intuitive approach and sought to determine whether basic syndromes of disturbance could be discovered by identifying clusters of correlated traits.

Hewitt and Jenkins analyzed 500 case records of children referred to the Michigan Child Guidance Institute because of behavior problems. The average age of this group was between 11 and 12, and the mean IQ was 94. Forty-five behavior items were rated for presence or absence and intercorrelated. This led to the delineation of three clusters of symptomatic traits:

1. "Overinhibited" behavior, characterized by seclusiveness, shyness, apathy, worrying, sensitiveness, and submissiveness;
2. "Unsocialized aggression," characterized by assaultive tendencies, starting fights, cruelty, defiance of authority, malicious mischief, and inadequate guilt feelings;
3. "Socialized delinquency," characterized by bad companions, gang activities, cooperative stealing, habitual truancy, absconding from home, and staying out late at night.

The more sophisticated methodology used by Hewitt and Jenkins appeared to confirm the hunches of the clinical workers: Paynter and Blanchard's "Personality difficulty" and Ackerson's "Personality problems" seemed to correspond to Hewitt and Jenkins' "Overinhibited" syndrome; the "Behavior difficulty" and "Conduct problems" categories of the earlier works were split into two syndromes—namely, "Unsocialized aggression" and "Socialized delinquency."

Hewitt and Jenkins also linked the three symptom clusters to etiological factors, as will be shown presently.

Use of factor analysis

With the application of factor analysis, further methodological refinement was introduced into research on child behavior. According to Harman (1967), "the principal concern of factor analysis is the resolution of a set of variables linearly in terms of . . . a small number of categories or 'factors' " (p. 4). . . . "A principal objective of factor analysis is to attain a parsimonious description of observed data" (p. 5).

Further analysis of Ackerson's data. Himmelweit (1952) selected 50 traits from the total number given by Ackerson and carried out a centroid analysis of the data for the boys in Ackerson's sample. The first two factors were a unipolar dimension of disturbed behavior which was called "Neuroticism" and a second dimension labeled "Introversion-Extraversion." Inspection of the results clearly indicates that the two factors corresponded to the categories established by Ackerson although they represented a different angle of rotation. Translated into Ackerson's terminology, Himmelweit found "Personality problems" to be disturbed behavior of an "introverted" nature (sensitive, seclusive, depressed) and "Conduct problems" to be impaired functioning of an "extraverted" type (stealing, truancy from home and school, destructive). Himmelweit's factorial study furnished statistical verification of Ackerson's work and thereby provided independent confirmation of his a priori approach to the grouping of behavior problems.

Application of distinction to "normal" children. Peterson (1961) broke new ground by identifying two basic syndromes of emotional disturbance in samples of "normal" children. As a first step, Peterson recorded the referral problems of 427 children representatively chosen from the records of a child guidance clinic. Elimination of redundant and very infrequently occurring referral problems resulted in a list of 58 items. Peterson then submitted his Problem Checklist to 28 teachers of normal children and asked them to rate their pupils on presence or absence of the problems. The subjects were 831 school children, divided into four age groups: a kindergarten sample ($N = 126$), a first and second grade sample ($N = 237$), a group of third and fourth graders ($N = 229$), and a fifth and sixth grade sample (N = 239). Peterson chose a school population rather than children undergoing treatment for judged disorders on the assumption that most such disorders were extremes of dimensions which ranged from healthy to disturbed.

Factor analysis revealed two major syndromes which Peterson called "Personality problem" and "Conduct problem."[1] Examination of the items indicates that the "Personality problem" syndrome (feelings of inferiority, lack of self-confidence, social withdrawal, proneness to become flustered) closely resembled the pattern that Hewitt and Jenkins had referred to as "Overinhibited" behavior while the "Conduct problem" syndrome (disobedience, disruptiveness, boisterousness, fighting) was similar to the category which Hewitt and Jenkins had labeled "Unsocialized aggression."

Bipolarity of the dimensions. Another study of elementary school pupils was headed by Schaefer who developed a Classroom Behavior Inventory designed to assess both desirable and undesirable behavior in the school setting (Schaefer, 1971; Schaefer & Aaronson, 1966; Schaefer, Droppleman, & Kalverboer, 1965). Three dimensions were found to account for most of the variability of the children's classroom functioning. The authors labeled these dimensions:

Factor I: Extroversion versus Introversion
Factor II: Love versus Hostility
Factor III: High versus Low Task Orientation

All three factors were found to be bipolar, i.e., each covered behavior ranging from healthy to disturbed. The negative pole of Factor I, apparently similar to Peterson's Personality problem factor, included items such as:

. . . Rarely joins in activities with others of his own accord

---

[1] We concur with Peterson in his dissatisfaction with the terminology; he stated, "Actually these terms, 'personality problem' and 'conduct problem,' are grossly inappropriate. Both problems are personality expressions, and both affect conduct. But the central meanings seem clear enough. In one case, impulses are expressed and society suffers; in the other case, impulses are evidently inhibited and the child suffers" (p. 206).

... Prefers working alone, leaves an activity if other children join him

... Becomes less effective and skillful in his work when being observed

The positive pole of Factor I covered the following kinds of behavior:

... Will readily talk with you about his activities, clothes, what he is doing

... Begins a conversation with another child who moves near him

... Is among the first to make a comment or ask a question about class activities

... Seeks others out to get them to interact with him, join in an activity with him

The negative pole of the Factor II dimension contained items highly suggestive of Peterson's Conduct problem factor. Examples are:

... Frequently gets in a temper if he can't have his way

... Is inclined to flare up if he's teased or picked on

... Gets impatient and unpleasant if he can't get what he wants when he wants it

... Gets annoyed for trivial reasons

The positive pole of Factor II represented behavior such as:

... Takes up for and tries to protect one whom others pick on

... Brings materials, equipment, cup of water, etc., to another

... Awaits his turn willingly

The third factor dimension, High versus Low Task Orientation, is not relevant in the present context and will be discussed in chapter 4.

The importance of Schaefer's work is that, by testing both desirable and undesirable classroom behavior, he provided evidence that each factor not only represented a syndrome of emotional disturbance but also extended along a continuum to a polar opposite in the realm of healthy functioning.

The line of inquiry was broadened in our laboratory to apply to children of preschool age, and the two dimensions which emerged from the factor analysis were designated Interest-Participation versus Apathy-Withdrawal and Cooperation-Compliance versus Anger-Defiance.

* * *

The foregoing survey has been selective rather than exhaustive; the aim was to single out the landmark studies which laid the groundwork for the development of the two-factor model of social-emotional functioning and to draw attention to key investigations which extended the range of application of the model: from clinical to normal populations and from disturbed to healthy modes of functioning. The extent to which increasingly sophisticated and complex analytic techniques have yielded parallel findings underscores the robustness and generality of the model.

The reader who is interested in other recent studies in which two principal diagnostic categories were isolated to describe childhood behavior or in which two major factors accounted for large amounts of behavior variability is referred to Bennett (1960), Conners (1970), Lewis (1954), Orpet and Meyers (1963), Patterson (1964), Peterson, Quay, and Cameron (1959), Ross, Lacy, and Parton (1965), and Rutter et al. (1970), among others.

Relationship of Child Behavior to Parental Behavior

There has been a paucity of research studies tracing the two fundamental syndromes of emotional impairment to one of their probable antecedents, i.e., the parent-child relationship.

Among the first to examine the effects of differing parental attitudes upon children with different types of maladjustment were Hewitt and Jenkins (1946). Corresponding to the three behavioral patterns—Overinhibited, Unsocialized aggression, and Socialized delinquency—Hewitt and Jenkins defined three "situational" patterns of family environment:

1. "Family repression," made up of items such as father's discipline inconsistent, father hypercritical, father or mother unsociable, mother dominating, sibling rivalry;

2. "Parental rejection," which included direct as well as indirect criteria of rejection, such as pregnancy unwanted by father or mother, post-delivery rejection by either parent, mother unwilling to accept parental role, mother sexually unconventional, mother openly hostile to child, loss of contact with both natural parents;

3. "Parental negligence and exposure to delinquent behavior," characterized by irregular home routine, lack of supervision, lax discipline, interior of home unkempt, mother shielding the child from (school, community) authorities, residence in a deteriorated urban area, sibling delinquency.

Hewitt and Jenkins also established a fourth pattern which is of less psychological interest since it involved chronic physical complaints, nervous system disorder, abnormal growth pattern, convulsions, auditory or speech defects. The pattern was called "Physical deficiency."

Tetrachoric correlations between the family situations and the behavior syndromes were calculated. As may be seen in Table 2.1, the authors found that both a repressive family environment

Table 2.1 Correlation of Situational Patterns with Behavior Syndromes

Situational patterns	Behavior syndromes		
	Overinhibited $N = 73$	Unsocialized aggression $N = 52$	Socialized delinquency $N = 70$
Family repression	.52	.10	−.12
Parental rejection	−.20	.48	.02
Parental negligence and exposure to delinquent behavior	−.17	.12	.63
Physical deficiency	.46	−.23	−.31
Family repression/physical deficiency combined	.73	.25	−.31

Note. — Adapted from Hewitt and Jenkins (1946), p. 68.

and physical disorders were likely to produce overinhibited behavior in the child.[2] A youngster with a background of parental rejection was apt to develop unsocialized aggressive ways of acting while parental neglect was strongly associated with subsequent socialized delinquent behavior on the part of the child.

Hewitt and Jenkins also postulated that for each type of behavior disorder a different type of treatment was appropriate.

* * *

Morris, Escoll, and Wexler (1956) made a systematic assessment of the parent-child relationship in the course of a follow-up study of children originally diagnosed as showing what the authors labeled "Aggressive behavior disorders." The sample consisted of 90 youngsters who had been admitted to the psychiatric division of the Pennsylvania Hospital for observation and treatment and who showed at least four of the following behavior traits: (a) repeated truancy from school or home, (b) stealing or purposeful lying, (c) cruelty, including marked teasing or bullying, (d) disobedience or defiance of authority, (e) marked restlessness or distractibility, (f) wanton destructiveness, and (g) severe temper tantrums when crossed. Further details about the sample will be presented with the follow-up studies in the next section of the chapter.

The authors found that, in a majority of the cases, there was open rejection of the child on the part of one or both parents. Parents were considered as openly rejecting if they met any one of the following criteria: (a) desertion of the child, (b) voluntary placement of the child in a foster home or institution, (c) removal of the child by decision of the court because the parents were "unfit", (d) open and constant expression of dislike for the child, or (e) marked preference for another sibling.

---

[2] When the two situational patterns were combined, the relationship to overinhibited behavior became even more pronounced.

The investigators concluded that "overt parental rejection, multiple parental figures, a high incidence of psychopathology in the immediate family, and open expression of feelings by the parents are the outstanding findings in the backgrounds of our children. Family behavior patterns seem to be very important; many of these children, brought up in environments where antisocial behavior was the rule rather than the exception, have continued to use aggressive antisocial behavior as their accustomed means of relating to people and situations" (p. 996).

* * *

Kohn and Rosman (1971) analyzed the mother-child relationship as part of a study on therapeutic intervention with disturbed children at several day care centers maintained by the New York City Department of Social Services. The youngsters were between 3- and 5-years old and had normal IQs. On the basis of teacher ratings of the children's functioning in the classroom, the authors selected for participation in the therapeutic intervention program 32 children who exhibited shy and inhibited behavior to an extreme degree (i.e., received very high scores on the dimension labeled Apathy-Withdrawal) and 32 children who manifested aggressive and dominating behavior to an extreme degree (i.e., were rated very high by their teachers on the dimension labeled Anger-Defiance).

Counselors attached to the day care centers conducted interviews with the mothers of each of the 64 youngsters to obtain data on the early mother-child relationship. The researchers developed two maternal behavior variables: (a) Maternal concern, rated on a 3-point scale ranging from "overprotection" = 1 to "rejection" = 3, and (b) Continuity of care, a pooled score ranging from 5 to 15, derived from the sum of five items dealing with the way the child was cared for during the first three years of life.

The correlations between the two maternal behavior variables and the children's scores on the two dimensions of functioning in the classroom indicated that the child high on Apathy-Withdrawal had experienced maternal overprotection and continuity of care whereas the child high on Anger-Defiance had had a rejecting mother and undependable maternal care.

Kohn and Rosman also found that the children tended to re-enact the mother-child pattern in the 1:1 relationship with the teacher during the course of the program of therapeutic intervention and concluded that the differential responses required different approaches in devising corrective emotional experiences.

* * *

Other clinical studies (Bannister & Ravdin, 1944; Bonney, 1941; Cummings, 1944; Levy, 1943; Lurie, 1970; Symonds, 1939) have yielded similar evidence about the genesis of the two syndrome patterns, or at least the concomitance between the behavior of parents and their offspring. But in view of the increased sophistication of theory and technique now available, it is unfortunate that no extensive research program has further focused on the connection between the parent-child relationship and the two-factor model of social-emotional functioning.

Long-Term Prognosis of Childhood Problems

Several teams of investigators have examined the life histories of emotionally disturbed individuals to discover what juvenile symptom patterns were precursors and predictive of pathology in adulthood. Researchers have either studied the developmental outcome of young patients who were diagnosed as emotionally impaired on one or the other syndrome (prospective approach), or they have taken adult patients as the point of departure and traced psychopathology back to the childhood behavior pattern (retrospective approach).[3]

Prospective approach

As noted above, Morris et al. (1956) worked with a sample of 90 acting-out patients at the Pennsylvania Hospital. The children

---

[3] We will comment in chapter 10 on the relative merits of the two approaches as part of a comprehensive evaluation of methods suitable for risk research.

were between the ages of 4 and 15 at intake (none had an IQ of less than 80, showed signs of organic brain damage, or were diagnosed as psychotic while in the hospital). The authors wanted to assess the "subsequent life adjustment" (p. 995) of the children. They were able to follow 66 subjects until age 18 and 48 subjects to age 30 or older. Of the 66, 13 became psychotic and were hospitalized with a diagnosis of schizophrenia; all but 1 have remained chronically ill. Over half of the group (39) never made an adequate social adjustment; 12 committed at least one crime of record although only one of the crimes involved violence or destruction. Only 14 patients eventually made an adequate adjustment.

The fact that almost 20% of the youngsters became chronically hospitalized schizophrenic adults is a sign of the extreme vulnerability of the overly aggressive child.

* * *

On the basis of clinic records, Morris, Soroker, and Burruss (1954) classified patients at the Dallas Child Guidance Clinic into three groups:

1. "Internal reactors": those who show predominantly shy, withdrawn, anxious, or fearful behavior, tend to develop neuroses, and bother themselves rather than others;

2. "External reactors": those who show aggressive or delinquent behavior, act out their difficulties, and bother other people;

3. "Mixed reactors": children with characteristics of each of the above groups.

The youngsters ranged in age from 3 to 15 when they were in treatment. Between 16 and 27 years later, the "Internal reactors" (N = 54) were followed up. On the basis of interview data, each subject was rated on a 3-point scale, as follows:

"Satisfactorily adjusted" = 1: those who are getting reasonable enjoyment, comfort, and fun out of living;

"Marginally adjusted" = 2: those who are not fulfilling their potential but are not in need of treatment; they are getting along but without much enjoyment or fun;

"Sick" = 3: those who are hospitalized or who have been hospitalized for mental or emotional disturbances; those who consider themselves ill enough to request help or whom the investigators deemed to require help.

In addition to these global assessments, ratings were made in such areas as self-evaluation, intimate relations, superficial relationships, and occupational adjustment.

Contrary to the authors' expectation that a large number of the "Internal reactors" would be schizophrenic as adults, the majority were relatively free of overt mental or emotional illness and were managing quite well. Almost two-thirds were classified as satisfactorily adjusted, one-third as marginally adjusted, and only two were sick: Of these, one was getting along with some difficulty in the community; the other was hospitalized with a diagnosis of schizophrenia.

The investigators concluded that, on the whole, extremely diffident children turned out to be average, normal adults in most respects: They continued to be quiet and retiring, were self-supporting and stable in their employment which tended to be sheltered; security in the job was emphasized rather than increasing opportunities and competitiveness.

* * *

A more extensive follow-up study was subsequently carried out by some of the same researchers (Michael, Morris, & Soroker, 1957). Their objective was to determine to what extent early diagnosis was predictive of later hospitalization.

All subjects had been patients at the Dallas Child Guidance Clinic when they were 9 years old. Their average IQ was 101, the range from 80 to 155. The time of follow-up was, on average, 26 years after the subjects had been seen at the clinic. The 606 children had been divided into three groups—"Introverts," "Extroverts," and "Ambiverts"—representing the same symptom clusters previously labeled Internal reactors, External reactors, and Mixed reactors.

The files of all Texas state mental institutions and V.A. hospitals were checked. The findings were: Only 1 of the 164

"Introverts" was hospitalized, with a diagnosis of schizophrenia; of 268 "Extroverts," 11 were found to have been hospitalized, 3 with a diagnosis of schizophrenia; of 174 "Ambiverts," 12 were found to have been hospitalized, 6 with schizophrenia.

These results were in line with the earlier findings suggesting that defiant and disruptive childhood behavior had potentially more serious consequences than passivity and submissiveness. The most potent indicator of poor prognosis appeared to be simultaneous disturbance on both symptom syndromes.

* * *

A very ambitious and incisive follow-up study of deviant children originally seen at the St. Louis Municipal Psychiatric Clinic was carried out by Robins (1966). Robins followed up 524 white children who had been patients at the clinic between 1924 and 1929 (children with an IQ below 80, youngsters who were referred but not examined, children seen for IQ testing only, and neglect and adoption cases were excluded from the study). Median age at referral was 13, and at follow-up the subjects were 30 years older. A non-referred normal control group was selected by matching year of birth, sex, and census tract.

Reason for referral was used as the basis for dividing the clinic population "into two gross categories, antisocial and non-antisocial. . . . It is a division that has been spontaneously paraphrased in almost every attempt to classify problem children" (p. 43). A partial list of reasons for referral for "antisocial" behavior included theft, burglary, robbery, truancy, running away or sleeping out, fighting, sexual perversion, and incorrigibility. By definition, all symptoms not classified as antisocial were called "non-antisocial" problems. Into this category were placed temper tantrums, irritability, depression, anxiety, restlessness, fears, school failures, inattention or daydreaming, etc.[4] By these criteria, 73% of the children came

[4] The list of non-antisocial problems seems to be more of a collection of left-overs than a unitary set of traits, as might have emerged from a factor analysis. The procedure appears to have been to include only the most obvious antisocial symptoms under that heading. The effect probably was to purify the antisocial syndrome but to incorporate some unwarranted and inappropriate items in the non-antisocial pattern.

Table 2.2 Reason for Referral and Later Diagnosis

Diagnosis	Patients referred for		
	Antisocial behavior $N = 314$	Non-antisocial behavior $N = 122$	Control group $N = 90$
No disease	16%	30%	52%
Sociopathic personality	28%	4%	2%
Alcoholism or drug addiction	8%	6%	2%
Psychosis	11%	11%	6%
Schizophrenia	5%	7%	2%
Neurosis	14%	33%	25%
Undiagnosed but sick	23%	16%	13%

Note. – Adapted from Robins (1966), p. 137.

to the attention of the clinic for antisocial behavior and 27%, for non-antisocial problems.

Robins developed a comprehensive set of measures of adult adjustment, only a few of which can be reported here. One outcome studied was diagnostic status. As may be seen in Table 2.2, the percentage of adults found to be emotionally healthy after 30 years was 52% for the control group, 30% for patients referred for non-antisocial behavior, and 16% for patients referred for antisocial behavior. When the percentage of persons with the relatively benign disease of "neurosis" is added to the percentage of individuals diagnosed as having "no disease," the following results emerge: 77% of the control subjects were classified as psychiatrically well or neurotic; 66% of the non-antisocial but only 30% of the antisocial subjects showed remission of symptoms or were neurotic. Clearly, children exhibiting antisocial problems were found to have a far worse prognosis than youngsters with non-antisocial symptoms.

Another outcome variable was arrest record. The data showed that antisocial behavior predicted to a generally high level of criminality: 71% of the male patients referred for antisocial behavior problems as compared to 30% of those referred for

Table 2.3 Number of Symptoms in Childhood and Diagnosis of
Sociopathic Personality as Adults

Number of juvenile symptoms	N	Diagnosis	
		Sociopathic personality	No disease
Antisocial symptoms			
Less than 3	115	4%	34%
3–5	93	15%	25%
6–7	71	25%	13%
8–9	75	29%	16%
10 or more	82	43%	5%
Non-antisocial symptoms			
Less than 2	91	22%	29%
2	62	16%	19%
3	73	26%	22%
4–5	100	21%	18%
6–8	83	22%	17%
9 or more	27	22%	4%

Note.—Adapted from Robins (1966), p. 142.

non-antisocial difficulties and 22% of the control group had
been arrested as adults for an offense other than a traffic charge.
The antisocial group also had been arrested more frequently and
for more serious crimes than the non-antisocial group.

The sociopathic personality syndrome was of major interest to
Robins. As expected, the group referred for antisocial behavior
produced the highest percentage of adult sociopaths: 28%, as
compared to 4% from the non-antisocial and 2% from the
control groups.

Robins then examined the extent to which the number of
juvenile symptoms was predictive of later diagnosis of
sociopathic personality.

The following trends may be observed in Table 2.3:

1. As the number of juvenile antisocial symptoms rose, there
was a decrease in the percentage of well adults and an increase
in the percentage of sociopaths.

2. As the number of juvenile non-antisocial symptoms

Table 2.4 Predicting Adult Antisocial Behavior in Non-Sociopaths from Number of Antisocial Symptoms in Childhood

Diagnosis other than sociopathic personality	Proportion with 5 or more adult antisocial symptoms when juvenile antisocial symptoms are totaled			
	Less than 6		6 or more	
	N	%	N	%
Schizophrenia	12	42	14	71
Chronic brain syndrome	3	33	7	71
Other psychoses	6	17	8	50
Alcoholism	9	33	24	83
Hysteria	9	33	11	55
Other neuroses	44	5	18	33
Undiagnosed	44	30	46	46
No disease	62	0	25	12

Note. – Adapted from Robins (1966), p. 148.

increased, there was also a decline in the percentage of healthy adults; however, there was no concomitant change in the percentage of sociopaths.

These results indicate that antisocial symptoms in children successfully forecast adult behavior involving a great deal of aggression and defiance of the social order; non-antisocial symptoms predict to emotional disturbance (as seen by the declining percentage of well adults) but not to disturbance which violates rules and norms.

Additional light on the long-range persistence of antisocial behavior was shed by Robins' findings involving adult diagnoses other than sociopathic personality. As displayed in Table 2.4, in every diagnostic category there was a direct relationship between juvenile and adult antisocial behavior: the higher the number of antisocial symptoms in childhood, the higher the percentage of adults with antisocial problems 30 years later.

* * *

A large-scale follow-up program was the Judge Baker Schizophrenia Project. A check of the names of almost 18,000 children who had been seen at the Judge Baker Child Guidance Center since it opened in 1917 against Massachusetts mental health records in 1965 disclosed 351 subjects who had been hospitalized and given quite definite diagnoses: schizophrenic (N = 196), alcoholic (N = 68), and impulsive character (N = 87). The investigators selected a comparison sample of 100 who were meeting reasonable work and social participation criteria for adult adjustment from among children also seen at the Guidance Center; the comparison sample was matched to the preschizophrenics on age, IQ, period when seen at the Center, etc.

The data have been analyzed from many perspectives and have given rise to a number of informative publications (see Fleming & Ricks, 1970; Nameche, Waring, & Ricks, 1964; Ricks & Berry, 1970; Ricks & Nameche, 1966; Waring & Ricks, 1965). We will concentrate on the report by Ricks and Berry and focus only on those findings which are germane to the present discussion—namely, the main symptom syndromes which the adult schizophrenics and impulsive characters had shown in childhood.

Ricks and Berry reported on 68 male schizophrenics, most of whom had been seen at the Guidance Center between the ages of 11 and 16. The investigators differentiated between a "chronic" group (individuals who were still hospitalized at the study's inception, N = 30) and a "released" group (persons whose hospitalization had been terminated at the time of follow-up, N = 38). The groups differed radically as to length of hospitalization; two-thirds of the chronics had spent more than 60% of their adult lives in mental hospitals.

Ricks and Berry found that "boys who later became chronic schizophrenics were of two distinct types which we shall label for later reference as: C1 'withdrawn' and C2 'delinquent.' C1 boys. . . showed withdrawal from school and community in conjunction with many other serious symptoms, including psychotic-like behavior, low self-esteem, obsessive thinking, and symptoms often associated with neurological impairment" (p. 39). Although shy and timid at school and in the community, these boys frequently showed "relatively uncontrolled acting-out behavior in the home—such as defiance of parents, tantrums, and disorganized destructive activity" (p. 39).

C2 boys "acted out extensively in the community and, in addition, showed many other symptoms, particularly low self-esteem and a second set of symptoms suggesting neurological impairment. . . . Their acting out in the community consisted largely of stealing, lying, truancy, and destructive activity. Rarely, however, did they physically molest others . . . . they generally were not aggressive or sadistic toward peers. Their home behavior was similar to the defiance and tantrums found among withdrawn chronics" (p. 39).

The released schizophrenics consisted to a large extent of two types which were designated R1 and R2. The R1 boys resembled the C1 youngsters in many respects: Their primary pattern was withdrawal; however, they gave less evidence of obsessive characteristics, psychotic-like symptoms, and symptoms associated with neurological impairment. The R2 boys manifested rebellious, defiant, and antisocial behavior, including deviant sexual practices, and, unlike the C2 boys, they acted out against their peers. Symptoms associated with neurological impairment were infrequent.

Thus, both syndromes (in conjunction with other symptoms) were found to be antecedents of schizophrenia. The results revealed that some children early manifested signs of detachment and regression and maintained the pattern of extreme apathy and withdrawal into adulthood. Other youngsters initially attempted to cope with the world by acting out but gave up protest and confrontation and then became reclusive and socially isolated. Of the latter group, those who showed their defiance in the home had a poorer prognosis than those who committed aggression toward their peers. Co-existence of the two dimensions in childhood, i.e., exhibiting different symptoms in different environments, was highly pathognomic of later psychopathology.

The impulsive characters ($N = 31$) showed antisocial behavior in both the home and the community. "Their patterns of acting-out behavior were specific to the group: one syndrome consisting of sexual deviance, stealing in the home, flagrant disobedience of both parents, and running away from home was characteristic only of future impulsive characters. They also tended to be defiant of community authorities and frequently engaged in destructive behavior in the community. Regarding social adjustment, capacity for empathic ties to peers was usually absent, and a high proportion had sadistic or sado-masochistic peer relationships" (p. 42). According to Ricks and Berry, "Compared with aggressive boys in other groups, those moving into character disorder showed many distinctive features" (p. 42); however, the exact nature of the differences between the antisocial behavior of the preschizophrenics and that of the impulsive characters is not made entirely clear by the authors.

Retrospective approach

In contrast to the studies cited above where researchers began with childhood pathology and assessed adult status, Watt and his associates (Watt, 1972, 1974; Watt, Stolorow, Lubensky, & McClelland, 1970) started with adult outcome and worked backwards. The objective was to reconstruct the childhood behavior patterns of hospital patients from their school records (a) to make comparisons with a matched control group who had made a socially adequate adjustment as adults, and (b) to look for sex differences in the behavior of preschizophrenic youngsters.

The investigators obtained from the Massachusetts Department of Mental Health a computer list containing the names of every patient between the ages of 15 and 34 who had been admitted to any public, private, or V.A. mental hospital between 1958 and 1965. The list was checked against the files of the public high school in a large residential and industrial suburb of Boston which Watt called "Maybury." Cumulative school records (i.e., for elementary school, junior high school, and high school) were located for 162 of the patients.

The initial data analysis (Watt et al., 1970) centered on 30 patients who had received a hospital diagnosis of schizophrenic, had attended Maybury High School, and had lived in Maybury at the time of first admission to the hospital. Their ages at first admission ranged from 18 to 31, with a mean of 23 years; median IQ was 104. For each preschizophrenic school record, three control records, matched for age, sex, parental social class, and race to the index case, were selected. None of the control group had ever been hospitalized for mental illness in Massachusetts before 1965 but it was not known whether all were still residing in the community.

Two types of measures were derived from the cumulative school records. One was based on a coding and scoring system for content analysis of the comments written annually by the teachers. The other consisted of a research assistant's global ratings of all comments on each total record for "conformity" (extent to which the youngster met the teacher's standards of appropriate classroom behavior, nature of his interpersonal relations with peers), "social participation" (extent to which the child took an active part in classroom discussions and activities as well as extracurricular activities), and "emotional stability" (extent to which the child exhibited self-control, social poise, personal security, and even temperament).

Watt et al. related their findings to two of the major patterns discovered by Hewitt and Jenkins—namely, Unsocialized aggression and Overinhibited behavior. They concluded, "Clearly, unsocialized aggression was the most prominent pattern of behavior in our preschizophrenic boys. They were more irritable, aggressive, negativistic, and defiant of authority than their matched controls... and they were inclined to be unpopular.... the preschizophrenic boys lacked scholastic motivation and dependability—further evidence of their defiance of authority and conventional social values at school.... By contrast to the boys, there was virtually no evidence of unsocialized aggression among the preschizophrenic girls" (pp. 652–653).

The girls were primarily quiet and introverted. The investigators stated, "The overinhibited pattern quite accurately describes the preschizophrenic girls in this study, as a group, although the statistical evidence is not nearly as strong as is the case for unsocialized aggression in the boys.... In short, whereas the preschizophrenic boys were undersocialized, the girls appear to be excessively socialized" (p. 653).

While recognizing that their sample was small, the researchers felt their data justified the conclusion that, as a group, children who became schizophrenic as adults behaved differently in school from other children and that the behavioral deviations were obvious enough for teachers to comment spontaneously on them on the school records. The pattern of maladjustment differed for boys and girls.

* * *

Although the studies reviewed varied in research approach, sample size, length of time interval between measurements, and kind and specificity of adult outcome criteria, the findings permit a number of generalizations: First, all of the studies point to the potential importance of the two major syndromes as forerunners of adult disorders. Second, a number of studies seem to support the view that the aggressive and dominating child has a worse long-term prognosis than the diffident and withdrawn youngster because he is (a) less likely to recover, (b) at greater risk of developing a neuropsychiatric disorder requiring hospitalization, and (c) more apt to run afoul of the law in later life. However, where extreme apathy and withdrawal is the marked syndrome or where it is seen together with antisocial behavior, the implications for risk of adult pathology are very serious. Third, there is a trend for emotional impairment to persist for long periods of time, with the bulk of the studies suggesting that antisocial behavior shows greater stability and, therefore, is a better predictor of future problems than inhibited functioning.

These comments are naturally qualified by the fact that they are based on research with clinical samples. To what extent the findings hold for the population at large remains to be tested.

Conclusions

The research on dimensions of childhood psychopathology has been fairly consistent in detecting two principal syndromes of emotional impairment, one characterized by apathy and passivity and the other, by aggressiveness and hostility. Both are low-competent ways of coping with the environment: the former by flight, the latter by fight.

The brief survey of the literature substantiated Peterson's (1961) contention that "the generality of these factors appears to be enormous . . . Considering all studies together, age has varied from early childhood to adolescence; problem status has varied from none, through clinic attendance, to incarceration for delinquency; data sources have varied from case history records, to standard ratings, to questionnaire responses; methods of factor extraction have varied from cluster inspection to centroid analysis; rotational methods have varied from none, through visual shifts to both orthogonal and oblique solutions, to analytic techniques. Through it all the factors have stayed the same" (p. 206).

We saw examples of the various labels that have been assigned to the same grouping of symptoms: Recessive behavior was called "Overinhibited" by Hewitt and Jenkins, "Introversion" by Schaefer and Aaronson, "Introverts" by Michael et al., and "Internal reactors" by Morris et al.; disruptive behavior traits were placed under the heading of "Unsocialized aggression" by Hewitt and Jenkins, "Hostility" by Schaefer and Aaronson, "Extroverts" by Michael et al., "External reactors" by Morris et al., and "antisocial" by Robins. The most common practice in research on childhood psychopathology has been to designate the two behavior patterns as problems of personality and conduct, respectively (Ackerson, Peterson), and the terms, "Personality problems" and "Conduct problems," will serve as reference points in the next chapter in which we will analyze the factors measured by our instruments and report on an empirical study designed to determine whether the various labels constituted alternate ways of describing the same two basic dimensions of functioning.

In some of the research that was described, a third major symptom cluster or factor emerged but the third dimension has varied from study to study. It would seem that the third factor depends on the social setting in which the data are gathered. Thus, in Hewitt and Jenkins' clinical sample, the third behavior pattern was "Socialized delinquency." In the Peterson and Schaefer studies, where the research setting was the classroom, the differentiation between unsocialized aggressive and socialized delinquent ways of acting did not appear, most likely because gang membership, absconding from home, etc., are not evident in the classroom. However, Schaefer and Aaronson found a third dimension related to task involvement, which is pertinent to a learning environment.

The literature review also showed that the constellations of behavior problems and symptoms subsumed under each of the major syndromes have different roots and different fates. To oversimplify in the interest of explicitness, children who are brought up in a family environment where they are intensely overprotected or severely controlled retreat from the world and take one of two routes through life: They either remain passive and retiring as adults and are able to function in the community or they withdraw even further into themselves and may require hospitalization. Youngsters who experience rejection and/or inconsistent treatment at home see the world as a hostile place and respond with defiance and attack; as they grow older, their aggressive ways may become intolerable to their family and/or community, and they may require institutionalization or incarceration.

More extensive research is needed on the association between the syndrome patterns and parental behavior. It is especially important to approach the inquiry with an open mind as to the flow of the cause-effect relationship. For example, parental overprotectiveness may produce a timid child but it is also possible that a fearful infant may evoke a greater-than-desirable amount of parental overindulgence.

As a final point, it should be recalled that Kohn and Rosman, as well as Hewitt and Jenkins, noted that different interventions are necessary for the two major syndromes of disturbance.

CHAPTER 3

Developing and Testing the Instruments

In this chapter we will trace the development of the two teacher rating instruments, the Symptom Checklist and the Social Competence Scale, which we used to assess the social-emotional functioning of children in a preschool setting and from which the two major syndromes of disturbance emerged after factor analysis (see chapter 1).

For the projected longitudinal study we also needed instruments that could assess the two dimensions of social-emotional functioning beyond the preschool period, in elementary school. Two options were open to us. We could either revise the Symptom Checklist and the Social Competence Scale to make them applicable to the functioning of elementary school children or we could use instruments already developed by other researchers. We tentatively embarked on the latter course primarily because we wanted to test the hypothesis that the conceptual similarity of the two fundamental dimensions, identified repeatedly in the literature in the past 50 years, was more than a superficial phenomenon: that the syndromes, although variously labeled according to each investigator's preferences, in fact referred to the same or at least very similar behavior patterns.

To obtain empirical evidence, we carried out a separate study in which we applied the Symptom Checklist and the Social Competence Scale and two other instruments, the Peterson Problem Checklist and the Schaefer Classroom Behavior Inventory (see chapter 2), to a group of children in day care and in elementary school. This research will also be described in the present chapter.

Development of Preschool Instruments

Symptom Checklist

The Symptom Checklist was designed to assess the presence or absence of behavior generally considered symptomatic of emotional impairment. In devising the instrument, we followed a procedure similar to that used by Peterson (1961); drawing on our own clinical experience as well as on recorded case material, we compiled a list of items descriptive of symptoms and problems which children, 3- to 5-years old, are likely to manifest in nursery school and day care settings.

An initial list of 90 items was pretested on 150 children in two day care centers. All items that were checked "sometimes" or "frequently" for 10% or more of the sample were retained; 32 items were eliminated, leaving a final list of 58 items.

Social Competence Scale

The Social Competence Scale was designed to assess the child's mastery of the preschool environment from the point of view of the child's interpersonal functioning. The Social Competence Scale was conceptually a more ambitious under-taking than the Symptom Checklist. In her survey of mental health concepts, Jahoda (1958) had made a strong case that absence of psychiatric symptoms was not necessarily synonymous with nor even an adequate criterion of psychological health. With the Social Competence Scale we wanted, therefore, to do more than differentiate between the presence or absence of pathology but to cover the entire spectrum from healthy to disturbed and thus also differentiate between various levels of healthy functioning.

In defining high and low social competence, we took the work of Chance (1959) as a starting point. Chance concluded that the way psychoanalytic theory describes the individual's manner of coping suggests at least two bipolar opposites—namely, active versus passive and friendly versus hostile. Chance hypothesized that these two dimensions are independent of each other and can be represented graphically as two lines perpendicular to each other, as shown in Figure 1. The combination of the two dimensions leads to four categories of interpersonal relationships: *positive active, positive passive, negative passive*, and *negative active*. In this framework, "Personality problems" can be viewed as falling into the negative passive section and "Conduct problems" as falling into the negative active sector.

With the four quadrants of Chance's model in mind, we prepared on initial pool of 200 items, to be rated on a 7-point frequency scale ranging from "always" to "never." Items which met Lorr, Klett, and McNair's (1963) criteria for scale construction were pretested on 45 children. Only items with sufficient interrater reliabilities ($p \leqslant .05$) were retained (reliabilities ranged from .35 to .78) although we intended ultimately to depend on the reliability of the factor scores and not on the reliability of individual items. At the conclusion of these various screening procedures, there remained a list of 90 items.

Methodology

The subjects were all children ($N = 407$) in six day care centers of the Division of Day Care of the New York City Department of Social Services. Three centers had a primarily white and three a primarily black population. The children

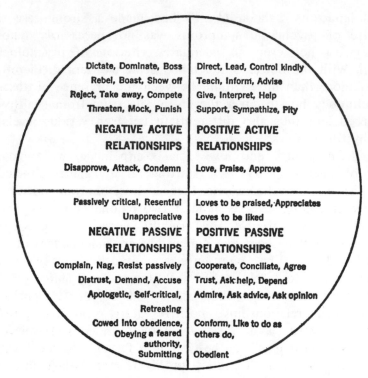

FIG. 1. "A System for Classifying Interpersonal Experiences,"
FAMILIES IN TREATMENT: *From the Viewpoint of the Patient,*
the Clinician and the Researcher by Erika Chance, Ph.D., (c)
1959 by Basic Books, Inc., Publishers, New York.

ranged in age from 36 to 70 months. The sample was divided
about equally between boys and girls. The racial and ethnic
composition of the group was 43% white, 40% black, 14%
Puerto Rican, and 3% Oriental. The children came from
predominantly lower- and lower-middle class backgrounds; about
49% of the families were broken, almost exclusively due to
father absence. Approximately 45% of the heads of household
had not completed high school, and about 50% of the families
had incomes of less than $5,000 per year.[5]

Each child was rated independently by the two full-time
teachers in the classroom on the 58-item Symptom Checklist
and the 90-item Social Competence Scale.

[5] This research was carried out in 1965.

To determine the major dimensions of the Symptom Checklist and the Social Competence Scale, each instrument was subjected to a factor analysis. In each case the first two rotated factors accounted for the major proportion of the total variance. On the Symptom Checklist, the first two of nine factors accounted for more than 50% of the total (communal) variance; on the Social Competence Scale, the first two of six factors accounted for 74% of the total (communal) variance. All but one of the remaining factors accounted for considerably less than 10% of the variance. Since the first two factors accounted for the major sources of the variation of both instruments, we decided to work with these two factors only.

Psychometric characteristics of the instruments

Factor dimensions of the Symptom Checklist. Both major factors of the Symptom Checklist were unipolar, measuring only varying degrees of disturbance. To convey what the factor dimensions represent, the five items with the highest loadings on each of the two factor dimensions are presented in Table 3.1. It may be seen that the Factor I items denoted passivity, withdrawal, and inhibition of functioning and were reminiscent of the "Personality problems" syndrome described in chapter 2. The Factor II items covered feelings of anger, defiance, and hostility and were strongly suggestive of the "Conduct problems" syndrome described in chapter 2.

Factor dimensions of the Social Competence Scale. Both major factors of the Social Competence Scale were bipolar, measuring the whole range from health to disturbance. To illustrate what is measured by these factor dimensions, the five items which showed the highest positive loadings and the five items which had the highest negative loadings on each factor are presented in Table 3.2. It is evident that the Factor I dimension reflected use of opportunities available in the classroom. The positive items indicated interest, assertiveness, involvement in classroom processes, and positive interactions with peers. The negative items indicated withdrawal from the opportunities of the classroom, lack of curiosity, passivity, and failure to elicit the cooperation of peers in carrying out activities. Thus, the negative

Table 3.1. Items with Highest Loadings on Factors I and II of the Symptom Checklist

Items	Factor	
	I	II
Part A: Highest loadings on Factor I		
Keeps to himself; remains aloof, distant	.85	.07
Fails to play with other children	.81	.04
Fails to take part in activities unless urged	.79	.11
Has a mournful, downcast expression, looks solemn, seldom smiles	.78	.06
Stares blankly into space	.73	.10
Part B: Highest loadings on Factor II		
Gets angry when interrupted at play by adult as part of normal routines (not punishment)	.01	.78
Treats other children with deliberate cruelty; bullies other children or hits or picks on them	.01	.76
Screams, bangs objects, etc., when angry, irritated, or frustrated	.03	.75
Fails to obey or follow instructions or directions of adult; "talks back" to adults	.10	.71
Gets angry or annoyed when addressed by adult, even in a friendly manner (not reprimand)	.14	.71

Note. – From "A Social Competence Scale and Symptom Checklist for the Preschool Child: Factor Dimensions, Their Cross-Instrument Generality, and Longitudinal Persistence" by M. Kohn and B. L. Rosman, *Developmental Psychology*, 1972, **6**, 435. Copyright 1972 by the American Psychological Association, Inc. Reprinted by permission.

Factor I dimension was conceptually similar to the "Personality problems" syndrome previously identified by other researchers.

Since Factor I was bipolar and since the negative pole seemed to suggest "Personality problems," we tentatively concluded that the cluster of symptoms designated as "Personality problems" was actually only one end of a continuum that ranged from apathy and withdrawal on the disturbed end to interest and participation on the healthy end.

Inspection of the Factor II items shows that they dealt with conforming to the rules and routines of the classroom. The

Table 3.2 Items with Highest Positive and Negative Loadings on Factors I and II of the Social Competence Scale

Items	Factor	
	I	II
Part A: Highest loadings on Factor I		
Child gets others interested in what he's doing	.83	.01
Child manifests interest in many and varied types of things	.83	−.12
Child displays enthusiasm about work or play	.82	−.21
Child can give ideas to other children as well as go along with their ideas	.82	−.20
Child is able to express his own desires or opinions in a group	.82	.07
Child has difficulty getting the attention of the group	−.80	.02
Child demonstrates little interest in things and activities of his environment	−.79	.13
Child fails to secure cooperation when he has to direct activities	−.77	.15
Child is at a loss without other children directing him or organizing activities for him	−.76	.07
Child spends time sitting around, looking around, or wandering around aimlessly	−.74	.26
Part B: Highest loadings on Factor II		
Child cooperates with rules and regulations	.28	.79
Child responds with immediate compliance to teacher's directions	.13	.73
Child is able to accept teacher's ideas and suggestions for play or ways of playing	.42	.64
Child makes transition from one activity to the next easily	.28	.62
Child puts things away carefully	.32	.60
Child disrupts activities of others	−.19	−.86
Child expresses open defiance against teacher's rules and regulations	−.08	−.84
Child is hostile and aggressive with other children (teases, taunts, bullies, etc.)	−.01	−.84
Child tries to prevent other children from carrying out routines	−.11	−.82
Child quarrels with other children	.00	−.80

Note.—From "A Social Competence Scale and Symptom Checklist for the Preschool Child: Factor Dimensions, Their Cross-Instrument Generality, and Longitudinal Persistence" by M. Kohn and B. L. Rosman, *Developmental Psychology*, 1972, 6, 434. Copyright 1972 by the American Psychological Association, Inc. Reprinted by permission.

positive items indicated living within the classroom structure, complying with the rules, and obeying the teacher. The negative items revealed rebelliousness, disruptiveness, and hostility and appeared to match the kinds of behavior labeled "Conduct problems" by previous investigators.

Since Factor II was bipolar and since the negative pole appeared to assess something aking to "Conduct problems," we concluded for this factor dimension also that the cluster of symptoms designated as "Conduct problems" was only one end of a continuum that ran from anger and defiance on the disturbed side to cooperation and compliance on the healthy side.

Interrater reliability. Scores for individual subjects on both Factors I and II of each instrument were obtained by summing the ratings of all items that were most highly loaded on the respective factor dimensions. The interrater correlations between pairs of teachers, as corrected by the Spearman-Brown formula, were .73 for both factor dimensions on the Symptom Checklist and .77 and .80 for Factors I and II, respectively, on the Social Competence Scale. These interrater reliabilities were deemed sufficiently high to make the instruments useful for the present research purpose.

Relationship between Factors I and II. In order to determine to what extent the two factors were independent or interrelated, the correlation between Symptom Checklist Factor I scores and Factor II scores was obtained; the correlation was low enough to indicate mutual independence (r = .18). On the Social Competence Scale, the correlation between the two sets of factor scores was .33, somewhat higher than desirable but low enough to suggest that the factors measured discriminably different dimensions of functioning.

Congruence between corresponding dimensions of the two instruments. Since the Factor I items of the Symptom Checklist as well as the items in the negative pole of Factor I of the Social Competence Scale all reflected apathy and lack of interest in classroom activities, it seemed reasonable to conclude that the two Factor I dimensions were highly congruent and should be strongly correlated. Similarly, because the Factor II items of the Symptom Checklist and the items in the negative pole of Factor

Table 3.3 Correlations between Symptom Checklist and Social Competence Scale Factors

Symptom Checklist	Social Competence Scale	
	Factor I	Factor II
Factor I	−.75	−.25
Factor II	−.13	−.79

Note. − *N* = 407.

High Symptom Checklist scores indicate disturbance; high Social Competence Scale scores indicate healthy functioning.

From "A Social Competence Scale and Symptom Checklist for the Preschool Child: Factor Dimensions, Their Cross-Instrument Generality, and Longitudinal Persistence" by M. Kohn and B. L. Rosman, *Developmental Psychology*, 1972, **6**, 435. Copyright 1972 by the American Psychological Association, Inc. Reprinted by permission.

II of the Social Competence Scale all depicted acting-out behavior in the classroom, we expected high congruence and substantial correlation between the two Factor II dimensions. At the same time, we anticipated no congruence between the non-corresponding factor dimensions of the two instruments.

A correlational analysis was carried out to test these assumptions. As may be seen Table 3.3, the corresponding factors were highly correlated ($r = -.75$ for Factors I; $r = -.79$ for Factors II) whereas r values between the non-corresponding factors were considerably lower (between $-.13$ and $-.25$).

Curvilinear relationship between corresponding dimensions of the two instruments. In addition to examining the linear relationship, we were interested in determining whether there was a curvilinear relationship between the dimensions. We

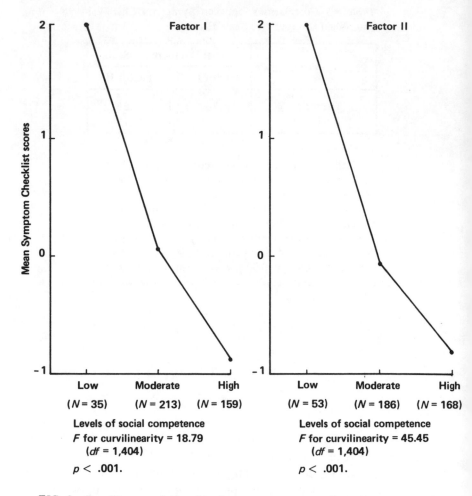

FIG. 2. Curvilinear relationship between corresponding dimensions of Symptom Checklist and Social Competence Scale.

hypothesized that Symptom Checklist scores would decrease sharply as Social Competence Scale scores increased from low to moderate levels of competent functioning; we expected no further drop in Symptom Checklist scores as Social Competence scores rose from moderate to high levels of functioning.

To test for curvilinearity of regression, a correlation ratio (*eta*) was computed by dividing the Social Competence Scale scores into three equal range intervals of "low," "moderate," and "high" for both Factor I and Factor II. The average Symptom Checklist score, expressed in z score units for each interval, was then calculated. Through analysis of variance of the Symptom score means, an F ratio for curvilinearity of 18.79 was obtained for Factor I, and an F ratio of 45.45 was obtained for Factor II, both significant at a level greater than .001. Figure 2 shows the plot of the Symptom Checklist versus Social Competence Scale scores.

As anticipated, for both factors, there was a steep decline in the Symptom scores between low and moderate levels of competence; contrary to expectations, the downward move continued, though at a significantly less precipitous rate, between moderate and high levels of competence. The results confirmed the fact that the Symptom Checklist made clear distinctions between different degrees of emotional impairment while the Social Competence Scale additionally discriminated among varying degrees of mental health.

The findings also supported Jahoda's contention that absence of pathology, at least as measured by gross behaviorally-evident symptoms, does not necessarily indicate optimum social-emotional functioning. While children who show a small number of overt symptoms are unlikely to be among the most disturbed, they are not necessarily among the healthiest.

Conclusion

On the basis of the psychometric data we decided that the Symptom Checklist and the Social Competence Scale could be used with confidence in the assessment of social-emotional functioning of children at the preschool level. The evidence also showed that personality functioning has crystallized sufficiently between the ages of 3 and 5 so that the two major syndrome patterns can be identified with considerable reliability.[6]

[6] In fact, there is moderate longitudinal stability on the factors between the ages of 3 and 5, indicating that by the time a child is 3 years old, these dimensions of personality functioning are already relatively stable attributes (see Kohn & Rosman, 1972b).

Congruence between Independently Developed Instruments

The two factor dimensions of the Kohn preschool instruments were designated Interest-Participation versus Apathy-Withdrawal and Cooperation-Compliance versus Anger-Defiance; Peterson (1961) used the more traditional nomenclature of Personality problems and Conduct problems; Schaefer and Aaronson (1966) referred to two of the three dimensions of the Classroom Behavior Inventory as Extroversion versus Introversion and Love versus Hostility. We tested the hypothesis that, in spite of the differences in terminology, the various instruments measured the same two basic dimensions of social-emotional functioning.

Methodology

The sample consisted of 287 boys attending public kindergarten and day care centers in New York City. The children ranged in age from 58 to 78 months. Half of the sample was black and half white. On the basis of Hollingshead's (1957) index, the subjects were selected in approximately equal numbers from three social class levels ranging from lower class to middle class. Black and white children were distributed evenly across social class levels.

The children were rated by their kindergarten and day care teachers on the Kohn Symptom Checklist, the Kohn Social Competence Scale, and the Schaefer Classroom Behavior Inventory. One year later, at the end of first grade, the youngsters were rated by their elementary school teacher on the Peterson Problem Checklist and the Schaefer Classroom Behavior Inventory.

The correlations between corresponding and non-corresponding factor dimensions were examined to determine whether the dimensions that had emerged from the preschool instruments were congruent with the dimensions of the elementary school instruments; specifically, whether a child who scored high on one of the two dimensions of the Kohn instruments also scored high on the corresponding dimension of the Peterson and Schaefer instruments and further, whether that score was unrelated to the rating on the non-corresponding dimension of each of the elementary school instruments.

Table 3.4 Correlations between Corresponding and Non-Corresponding Factor Scores Across Instruments

Factors	*r*
Part A: Preschool (*N* = 287)	
Corresponding factors	
Symptom Checklist Factor I vs. Schaefer Factor I	−.81**
Social Competence Factor I vs. Schaefer Factor I	+.80**
Symptom Checklist Factor I vs. Social Competence Factor I	−.72**
Symptom Checklist Factor II vs. Schaefer Factor II	−.76**
Social Competence Factor II vs. Schaefer Factor II	+.83**
Symptom Checklist Factor II vs. Social Competence Factor II	−.86**
Non-corresponding factors	
Symptom Checklist Factor I vs. Schaefer Factor II	−.24**
Symptom Checklist Factor II vs. Schaefer Factor I	−.03
Social Competence Factor I vs. Schaefer Factor II	+.48**
Social Competence Factor II vs. Schaefer Factor I	+.15**
Symptom Checklist Factor I vs. Social Competence Factor II	−.17**
Symptom Checklist Factor II vs. Social Competence Factor I	−.31**
Part B: First grade (*N* = 271)	
Corresponding factors	
Peterson Factor I vs. Schaefer Factor I	−.64**
Peterson Factor II vs. Schaefer Factor II	−.76**
Non-corresponding factors	
Peterson Factor I vs. Schaefer Factor II	−.42**
Peterson Factor II vs. Schaefer Factor I	−.12*

Note.—On the Symptom Checklist and the Peterson Problem Checklist, high scores = disturbance; on the Social Competence Scale and the Schaefer Classroom Behavior Inventory, high scores = health.

  *$p \leqslant .05$.
  **$p \leqslant .01$.

Results

The correlations between the corresponding and non-corresponding factor dimensions are presented in Table 3.4. It is apparent that at the preschool level the correlations between corresponding factors of the Kohn instruments and the Schaefer Classroom Behavior Inventory were high (median *r* = .78), and the correlations between non-corresponding factors were modest (median *r* = .21).

The same pattern was found at the first grade level for the correlations between corresponding and non-corresponding factors of the Peterson Problem Checklist and the Schaefer Classroom Behavior Inventory.

In other words, we may infer that (a) with respect to the corresponding dimensions: At the disturbed end of the continuum, children rated high on Apathy-Withdrawal on the Symptom Checklist and the Social Competence Scale scored high on Peterson's Personality problems and high on the Introversion pole of Schaefer's Extroversion versus Introversion dimension; youngsters rated high on Anger-Defiance on the Kohn instruments had high scores on Peterson's Conduct problems and on Hostility on Schaefer's Love versus Hostility dimension. Conversely, at the healthy end of the continuum, children who were high on Interest-Participation and Cooperation-Compliance on the Social Competence Scale were also high on Extroversion and Love, respectively, on the Schaefer instrument.

Thus, we had demonstrated empirically that, regardless of labels, corresponding factors from four different instruments developed by three different research teams in three different laboratories measured essentially the same behavior.

(b) With respect to the non-corresponding dimensions: The scores on the Apathy-Withdrawal—Personality problems—Introversion dimension showed only modest relationships to those on the Anger-Defiance—Conduct problems—Hostility dimension although a few of the correlations were somewhat higher than desirable (see particularly Social Competence Factor I versus Schaefer Factor II and Peterson Factor I versus Schaefer Factor II). On the whole, the data indicated that the two factor dimensions of each instrument were relatively independent of each other, measuring discriminably different behavior traits.

Conclusion

The pattern of correlations among the various research instruments further underscored our conviction that the generality of the two major syndromes of disturbance is, as Peterson put it, "enormous." With the hypothesis about the congruence between the instruments confirmed, we concluded that little would be lost in the way of continuity if we assessed social-emotional functioning with the Kohn Symptom Checklist and the Kohn Social Competence Scale at the preschool level and with the Peterson Problem Checklist and the Schaefer Classroom Behavior Inventory during the elementary school phase of the longitudinal study.

Terminology for the Longitudinal Study

We made two decisions regarding the labeling of the factor dimensions:

1. To adopt the Kohn designations of Interest-Participation versus Apathy-Withdrawal for Factor I and Cooperation-Compliance versus Anger-Defiance for Factor II in reporting the longitudinal study. This was not intended to imply the superiority of these terms over those used by Peterson and Schaefer but was done rather (a) in the interest of consistency, and (b) as a reflection of our basic assumption about the factor scores. We believed that the dimensions do not necessarily measure invariant attributes of the personality. All that we can meaningfully say is that we are measuring a child's behavior in a given setting—namely, the classroom. Whether his behavior in the classroom has some degree of stability over time and/or is characteristic of his behavior in other settings has yet to be determined.

2. To shorten the Kohn designations to Apathy-Withdrawal and Anger-Defiance, where feasible. This was done solely for the sake of convenience and did not imply that we were only concerned with pathology.

CHAPTER 4
Methodology of the Study

The present study was conceived as a five-year longitudinal project: At the outset of the study in the fall of 1967, the children were attending public day care centers in New York City, and they were followed until they completed the fourth grade of elementary school. In this chapter the methods employed in the study and their rationale will be described.

As a first step, Miss Muriel Katz, Director of the Division of Day Care of the New York City Department of Social Services, wrote a letter to the directors of the 92 public day care centers under the Division's jurisdiction to inform them about the proposed study and to enlist their cooperation. About two months later, in November 1967, we contacted the director of every day care center to discuss the project with her and, with her assistance, we chose a randomly selected sample of children from her classroom lists to be the subjects of the study. Two day care centers declined to participate because of previous commitments to other research projects.

Subjects

The subjects consisted of a 20% random sample (N = 1,232) of the day care population. The children ranged in age from 3 to almost 6 and were divided into three age groups or cohorts, as follows: Cohort A (N = 428), eligible for first grade in September 1968 (age range, 59–70 months); Cohort B (N = 468), eligible for first grade in September 1969 (age range, 47–58 months); and Cohort C (N = 336), eligible for first grade in September 1970 (age range, 35–46 months).

The sample was divided almost equally between boys and girls. The children came from lower-, lower-middle, and middle-class families, slightly more than 50% of which were one-parent households. Fifty-six percent of the youngsters were black, 27% were white, and 16% were Puerto Rican. Of the children's mothers, 45% had not completed high school; on the other hand, 12% had attended college. Nine percent of the families had an annual income below $3,000; approximately 45% had incomes below $5,000. Nineteen percent of the families received public assistance. Thus, the socioeconomic range was somewhat restricted compared to the population of children at large.

Major Variables

The study dealt with three classes of variables: demographic, emotional impairment, and academic attainment.

Demographic variables

Demographic variables define the individual's position in the social system and his relationship to the social order. The number of potentially fruitful variables is enormous. In the present study we were guided by the approach of the Midtown

Manhattan Project (Srole et al., 1962); the authors stated: "The only practical alternative is purposively to select from this universe a few theoretically promising (and technically research-able) landmarks for exploration" (p. 17).

In the present study we utilized five variables which can be divided into three categories:

1. Bio-social variables, covering given attributes which are socially significant—namely, *age* and *sex*.

2. Sociocultural variables, which define the individual's place in the social order and his socially-patterned interaction within and between groups—namely, *race-ethnicity* (i.e., white, black, or Puerto Rican) and *social class*, as measured by mother's education. Education and occupation are frequently used as indices of social class (see Hollingshead's two-factor system, 1957). Since in approximately half of the households there was no father, mother's education was the social class criterion that could be applied with the least ambiguity to our sample. Kagan and Moss (1962) have pointed out: "The predictive power of parental educational level rests on its implications for the total life experiences of the child" (p. 153).

3. Family attributes, which index the characteristics of the primary group to which the individual belongs—namely, *family intactness*. There is considerable consensus among social scientists that family cohesion and the stability of parental relationships play an important role in the healthy development of children. As Srole et al. (1962) noted, "The potential implications of . . . interparental fracture for the personality of the growing child would seem to be considerable" (p. 196). In the present study we used "family intactness" as an easily accessible though far from perfect measure of this aspect of family life.[7]

----

[7]To determine selectivity of attrition, which will be discussed presently, the following variables pertaining to the family were also considered: number of siblings, occupational level of head of household, family income, welfare status, and family stability (see Table 4.5).

Preschool measures of emotional impairment

There were two kinds of preschool variables:

1. The two syndromes of *Apathy-Withdrawal* and *Anger-Defiance* which were assessed by means of the two Kohn instruments, the Symptom Checklist and the Social Competence Scale, described in chapter 3. It will be recalled that these instruments measured not only type of disturbance but also severity of disturbance on each syndrome. The instruments were revised slightly for the present study because the magnitude of the project (90 day care centers located throughout the City of New York) made it impossible to give individualized rating instructions to the teachers and clear up ambiguities in face-to-face contacts with them. Since almost all communication was by mail, the instruments had to be self-administering. To achieve this objective, 15 pairs of teachers in 15 classrooms were asked to complete the instruments. The research staff analyzed discrepancies between pairs of teachers and re-wrote items to minimize ambiguities and sources of alternative interpretations. The revised Symptom Checklist had 49 items, and the revised Social Competence Scale had 73 items. A set of written instructions was formulated.

2. Two teacher ratings of overall functioning in the classroom—namely, *Global Impairment* and *Referral* for psychiatric, psychological, or remedial help. These unidimensional scales measured severity of emotional impairment without regard to the nature of the impairment and were of a type frequently employed in previous studies (cf. Bower, 1969, p. 46, 72 ff). When used as dependent variables, these global ratings were seen as criterion measures which provided one approach to determining the validity of Apathy-Withdrawal and Anger-Defiance as indicators of pathology.

Global Impairment was measured on a 3-point scale, as follows:

"Well functioning" = 1: A child who gets along well with teachers and other children, participates with interest in activities, and is able to accomplish the tasks that are usually mastered by children his age. He appears alert, self-sufficient, friendly, and unafraid.

"Moderately-well functioning" = 2: A child who manages fairly adequately but shows some difficulty in one or several areas. He might be characterized as a child for whom growing up represents something of a struggle and who is not as happy as he might be.

"Poorly functioning" = 3: A child who has more difficulty than most youngsters his age in adjusting to the school setting. Poor functioning might manifest itself in many different ways such as problems in getting along with teachers and other adults, difficulties in relating to other children, and/or lack of ability to sustain any prolonged interest in the activities of the classroom. In short, compared to others in the group, the child exhibits signs of disturbance.

On the Referral rating, the teacher indicated whether (a) the child was receiving psychiatric or psychological treatment or referral for such treatment was indicated, or (b) the child was receiving remedial or special (non-medical) help or referral for remedial help was indicated, or (c) no referral was necessary. This information was coded on a 2-point scale: "in treatment or referral necessary" = 1; "no treatment or referral necessary" = 0.

The ability of teachers to detect children's emotional problems and the congruence and divergence between the perceptions of teachers and clinicians have been the subject of serious study since the 1920's. Wickman (1928) in his pioneering work asked teachers to rate the seriousness of children's current problems and asked mental health specialists to rate the seriousness of the consequences of the problems to the children's future functioning. Given the lack of comparability in what the two groups were assessing, it was not surprising that there was little congruence between the ratings of the two groups. Nevertheless, many people concluded from Wickman's study that teachers and mental health specialists did not perceive children's behavior from the same point of view. When Mitchell (1942) changed the administrative procedure so that both groups received the same instructions, he obtained a correlation of .70 between the teachers and the mental hygienists.

A direct test of the validity of teachers' global ratings was carried out by Bower (1969). A criterion group of emotionally disturbed fourth, fifth, and sixth grade children from several California school districts with well-developed psychological and psychiatric services was selected by psychologists, guidance counselors, and other mental health specialists. The teachers did not know who the children in the criterion group were. Among other procedures, they rated all children in their classroom on a 3-point scale of adjustment ("among the best" = 1; "average" = 2; "among the poorest" = 3). Eighty-seven percent of the children in the criterion group were rated "among the poorest."

The fact that teachers are able to select with a marked degree of accuracy children in need of psychological or psychiatric treatment is borne out by adult follow-up of such children. Fitzsimmons (1958) followed up 158 pupils referred for "intensive study" by their teachers. A comparison of the original case history material with the assessment made 15 years later showed that the teachers had been able to spot quite accurately those children who were to experience severe emotional difficulties in later life.

It is important to emphasize that Global Impairment and Referral encompassed practically everything that a teacher takes into account in arriving at a judgment of disturbance. We will return to this point in subsequent chapters when we will contrast the global ratings with the specific syndromes, Apathy-Withdrawal and Anger-Defiance, to determine whether the syndromes also are comprehensive measures covering a relatively large part of terrain labeled emotional disturbance in childhood.

Elementary school measures of emotional impairment

The elementary school variables were similar to the preschool variables—namely, syndromes of disturbance and global ratings:

1. *Apathy-Withdrawal* and *Anger-Defiance* were assessed by means of the Peterson Problem Checklist and the Schaefer Classroom Behavior Inventory. We felt justified in using these two instruments for elementary school assessment since (a) they

were specifically designed for this age group, and (b) we had previously determined (see chapter 3) that they measured the same two patterns of disturbance as the preschool instruments.

In addition, we introduced a third dimension—namely, *High versus Low Task Orientation*, which is measured by the Schaefer Classroom Behavior Inventory. Like the other two variables which emerged from Schaefer's factor analysis of his instrument (see chapter 2), this dimension is bipolar. At the healthy end, High Task Orientation indicates the extent to which the child focuses his attention, is able to concentrate, to become absorbed in activities, and to persevere in the face of difficulties. Examples of items are:

... Centers his attention on what he is doing and nothing seems to distract him
... If one effort to do a job is unsuccessful, will try again
... Gives undivided attention to a project or activity that catches his interest
... Nearly always sticks to tasks until they are finished

The disturbed end of the dimension, Low Task Orientation, indicates hyperactivity, distractibility, short attention span, and low motivation to "stick to" or complete tasks and activities, as illustrated by these items:

... Frequently is twisting, turning or getting up from his chair
... Often does not complete a task or errand because other things have captured his attention
... Any outside activity or noise can distract his attention from what the teacher is saying

Anger-Defiance and Low Task Orientation overlap. They both assess the child's ability to function within rules, limits, and norms; however, the first evaluates the youngster's ability to operate in an orderly way in the classroom as a whole whereas the second measures his ability to organize himself around specific tasks. We were interested to see whether the two patterns would generate differential predictions regarding scholastic achievement and longitudinal persistence of emotional impairment.

Task orientation is an important, though relatively neglected, area of child development. One of the first developmental psychologists to draw attention to its importance was Charlotte Buehler (1935). Buehler believed that work attitude and task set developed in several stages: Toward the end of the first year of life, the child is no longer solely concerned with his own movements but pays attention to the nature of material and becomes aware of the effects of his action upon it. From the second to the sixth year, the child's treatment of various materials is not only increasingly specialized but his manipulative techniques become more and more adapted to the nature of the materials. The willful, egocentric, unplanned attack of the younger child is gradually replaced by the carefully planned application of skill.

At about 1½ years of age, the child becomes aware of unintentional products of his play as, e.g., when he accidentally places one block on another. In time this activity will become intentional, leading to satisfaction and pride in accomplishment as well as to work, i.e., the systematic effort to create a new entity. Buehler noted: "It is obvious that this transition from activity that is primarily concerned with the establishment of movement patterns, to activity that utilizes these patterns only as a means to a constructive end is of far-reaching significance" (p. 83). During the preschool period, the child's "work" activity is primarily symbolic; from about the age of 5 on, the child's productions become realistic rather than "make-believe." Buehler considered this intentional work-play and striving towards a product as a crucial developmental step and as the foundation and major prerequisite of school success.

In a study of first grade children who failed, Danziger (1933) found that 80% failed because they had not developed a work attitude in their games before entering school. She reported that only 6% of the failures were in one subject, 50% in two, and 44% in three subjects. Failure in first grade was seldom due to the child's inability to perform successfully in a given subject nor to any particular deficiencies but rather to a general disability that manifested itself whenever the child attempted to undertake anything.

Independently, Lindeman and Ross (1955) came to similar conclusions; they found that preschool children's task involvement, assessed in a doll play situation, was significantly related to the children's later adjustment in kindergarten and first grade. In recent years the concept of task orientation has aroused renewed interest as a focal measure of the child's psychological development (see Heinicke, Friedman, Prescott, Puncel, & Sale, 1973).

2. *Global Impairment* and *Referral* for psychiatric, psychological, or remedial help were designed to measure the children's overall functioning in the classroom. The scales used in preschool were again utilized in elementary school.

Measures of academic attainment

In day care the teachers rated the children on *Verbal Fluency*. Strictly speaking, this was not an achievement measure but was rather designed to yield a rough measure of intelligence. Previous research had shown verbal ability to be a salient component of cognitive functioning (Bloom, 1964; Kohn & Cohen, 1975; Kohn & Rosman, 1973a). The definition of the scale points were: "superior" = 1; "average" = 2; "poor" = 3; "minimal or no speech" = 4.

Achievement in elementary school was evaluated by a variety of measures:

.1. *Metropolitan School Readiness Test.* This test used to be administered by the New York City Board of Education one month after the beginning of the school year.

2. *Metropolitan Achievement Tests.* These tests are administered routinely by the New York City Board of Education to all children attending the New York City public schools and are machine-scored by an independent data processing firm. There are two Verbal subtests, Work Knowledge and Reading, administered every year beginning with grade 2, and three Arithmetic subtests, Mathematics Concepts, Mathematics Problem Solving, and Mathematics Computation, administered in grade 3.

Children attending parochial or private schools were tested by members of the research staff.

3. *Academic Standing.* Beginning with first grade, the teacher was asked to assess the child's academic performance relative to that of the rest of the class on a 3-point scale ranging from "in the lowest third" = 1 to "in the highest third" = 3.

4. *Verbal Fluency.* A rating was made every year, employing the same scale as the one used in day care.

5. *Grade Placement.* According to Board of Education policy, date of birth was the basis for determining the grade in which a child should be. As noted at the beginning of the chapter, Cohort A children were eligible for first grade in September 1968; Cohort B children, one year later; and Cohort C children, two years later.

Beginning with second grade and every year thereafter, a child received a Grade Placement score, as follows: A child who skipped one or more grades received a score of +1 or +2, depending on the number of grades he skipped; a child who was in the appropriate grade level was given a score of 0; a child who was left behind received a score of −1 or −2, depending on the number of grades he was held back.

6. *Level Within Grade.* On the final rating occasion, the teacher was asked to record whether the class which the child was attending was, relative to the other classes at the same grade level, "among the brightest" = 3; "middle" = 2; "among the slowest" = 1.

Summary

To sum up, the major variables of the present study were:

Demographic variables:
    Age
    Sex
    Race-ethnicity
    Social class
    Family intactness
Preschool measures of emotional impairment:
    Apathy-Withdrawal
    Anger-Defiance
    Global Impairment
    Referral

Elementary school measures of emotional impairment:
Apathy-Withdrawal
Anger-Defiance
Low Task Orientation
Global Impairment
Referral
Measures of academic attainment:
Preschool
Verbal Fluency
Elementary school
Metropolitan School Readiness Test
Verbal Achievement (Metropolitan Achievement Tests)
Arithmetic Achievement (Metropolitan Achievement Tests)
Academic Standing
Verbal Fluency
Grade Placement
Level Within Grade

Procedures

Data were collected at regular intervals over the five-year period of the study. Since the children were in different age groups (cohorts) at the onset of the study, they were followed for varying periods in day care and elementary school. Cohort A (age 5) was followed for one year in day care and for four years in elementary school (through the fourth grade). Cohorts B and C (ages 4 and 3, respectively) were studied for two years in day care; Cohort B was followed for three years in elementary school (through third grade) and Cohort C, for two years (through second grade). The cohort to which the child belonged was determined by his date of birth; if, during elementary school, he skipped or had to repeat a grade, he still remained in the same cohort.

Demographic data

At the beginning of the study in November 1967, counselors attached to the day care centers completed a Background Data

Form on each child. An interview was held with the child's parents (usually the mother), and at the same time parental consent for the child's participation in the study was obtained. Twelve parents declined to give consent, and data collection for their children was discontinued.

Preschool social-emotional functioning

Data were collected four times using the two Kohn instruments, Symptom Checklist and Social Competence Scale, and the two global measures, Global Impairment and Referral. All but Referral were completed independently by both full-time teachers in the classroom; Referral was completed by the head teachers only since it was generally their responsibility to bring referrals to the attention of the day care center director. The first rating occasion (Rating 1) was in November 1967; the second, six months later (Rating 2). For Cohorts B and C, still in day care, data were obtained at two subsequent six-month intervals.

The revised Symptom Checklist and Social Competence Scale were analyzed to determine (a) interrater reliabilities to gauge the trustworthiness of the instruments, and (b) cross-instrument correlations between corresponding and non-corresponding factors to establish the congruence of the corresponding dimensions and the relative independence of the non-corresponding dimensions. In addition, various data pooling procedures were instituted in order to enhance the reliability of the measurements and simplify the data analysis.

Psychometric characteristics. The psychometric characteristics of the Symptom Checklist and the Social Competence Scale are presented in Table 4.1. Part A of the table shows the interrater reliabilities (Spearman-Brown corrected) at each of the four rating occasions. The reliabilities ranged from .53 to .83, with the median reliability $r = .75$, and were sufficiently high to warrant use of the instruments.

Part B of the table contains the cross-instrument correlations between corresponding and non-corresponding factor dimensions. For these correlations the corresponding scores from the two teachers rating the same child were summed (i.e., Symptom

Table 4.1 Psychometric Characteristics of Preschool Instruments at the Four Rating Occasions

Factors	Rating 1 N = 1,232	Rating 2 N = 1,074	Rating 3 N = 556	Rating 4 N = 605
Part A: Estimated interrater reliabilities (Spearman-Brown corrected)				
Symptom Checklist Factor I	.69	.53	.60	.65
Symptom Checklist Factor II	.77	.69	.78	.83
Social Competence Scale Factor I	.74	.71	.70	.79
Social Competence Scale Factor II	.76	.77	.76	.82
Part B: Cross-instrument correlations of pooled teacher scores				
Corresponding factors				
Symptom Checklist I vs. Social Competence Scale I	−.74	−.79	−.69	−.70
Symptom Checklist II vs. Social Competence Scale II	−.82	−.81	−.81	−.84
Non-corresponding factors				
Symptom Checklist I vs. Social Competence Scale II	−.22	−.24	−.25	−.25
Symptom Checklist II vs. Social Competence Scale I	−.26	−.29	−.36	−.38
Part C: Estimated reliabilities of pooled instrument scores				
Pooled Instrument Factor I	.83	.76	.79	.84
Pooled Instrument Factor II	.83	.84	.87	.90

Note.—On the Symptom Checklist and pooled instrument scores, high scores = disturbance; on the Social Competence Scale, high scores = health.

The large drop in *N*'s between Rating 2 and Rating 3 is due to the fact that Cohort A, the first group to enter elementary school, is not included in the table after Rating 2.

For total subjects rated by the head teacher and the assistant teacher, *N* = 1,110, 917, 496, and 559 for Ratings 1, 2, 3, and 4, respectively. Because of job vacancies, approximately 10% of the children were rated by only one teacher. In order to keep measures comparable, the single teacher scores were doubled in these cases. All reliability coefficients are based on cases in which both teachers rated the child.

Adapted from Kohn and Rosman (1972b), p. 437.

Checklist Factor I was based on the ratings made by both full-time teachers in the classroom, and a similar procedure was followed for each of the other factors). It may be seen that corresponding factor dimensions of the two instruments were highly congruent: The correlations varied between −.69 and −.84, with the median $r = -.78$. The correlations between non-corresponding factors ranged from −.22 to −.38, with the median $r = -.26$, and were sufficiently low to confirm the relative independence of the two dimensions of social-emotional functioning.[8]

[8] Similar results based on a sample of 407 subjects were presented in the previous chapter (see Table 3.3). Comparison of the above data with those in chapter 3 reveals that the revision of the instruments did not change the basic measurement characteristics of the instruments.

In view of the high correlations between the corresponding factor dimensions of the Symptom Checklist and the Social Competence Scale and for the purpose of further increasing the reliability of measurement, the corresponding factor scores from the two instruments were pooled. The procedure was as follows: Using the scores from the first rating occasion (Rating 1) as the standardization base, the pooled teachers' raw scores were converted to standard scores. Since the instruments have scores running in opposite directions (high Symptom scores indicate disturbance; high Competence scores indicate health), the signs of the Social Competence Scale scores were reversed. The standardized Factor I scores from the Symptom Checklist were then added to the standardized Factor I scores from the Social Competence Scale to yield a pooled instrument Factor I score for each child at each rating occasion. A comparable procedure was followed to obtain a pooled instrument Factor II score for each child at each rating occasion. High pooled instrument scores indicated disturbance.

The reliabilities of the pooled instrument scores are presented in Part C of Table 4.1. The reliabilities were satisfactorily high, varying between .76 and .90, with a median r of .84.

Pooling of Global Impairment scores. For each of the four rating occasions, the ratings made by the two full-time teachers were pooled. The pooled score ratings ranged from 2 to 6, and the interrater reliability of the pooled ratings (Spearman-Brown corrected) was .82. The figure was high enough to make the measure useful for our purposes.

Averaging across rating occasions. In order to obtain maximally stable measures for the longitudinal predictions, the pooled instrument scores, the pooled Global Impairment scores, and the Referral ratings made by the head teachers, were each averaged over the preschool rating occasions.

Elementary school social-emotional functioning

Toward the end of each school year, in late April or early May, the children were rated by their teacher on the Peterson Problem Checklist and the Schaefer Classroom Behavior Inventory as well as on the two measures of overall functioning, Global Impairment and Referral.

The psychometric characteristics of the Peterson Problem Checklist and the Schaefer Classroom Behavior Inventory were examined, specifically, the within-instrument and cross-instrument correlations of the corresponding and non-corresponding factor dimensions. In addition to determining the extent to which the two corresponding factors were congruent and the two non-corresponding factors independent of each other, we were interested in the relationship of Schaefer's Factor III, Task Orientation, to the other Schaefer factors and to the two Peterson dimensions.

Interrater reliabilities could not be calculated since each child was rated by only one teacher. Peterson (1961) reported interrater reliabilities of .77 and .75 for Factors I and II, respectively. Schaefer, Droppleman, and Kalverboer (1965) reported a modest median interrater correlation of .50 for the 12 subscales of which the Classroom Behavior Inventory is composed. However, since each of the Schaefer factor dimensions is measured by four subscales, the reliability with which each of the factor dimensions is measured is considerably higher ($r = .80$, estimated by the Spearman-Brown formula).

Within-instrument correlations. Peterson (1961) found the intercorrelation between his Factor I and II to be .18. Schaefer and Aaronson (1966) reported the following correlations: Factor I versus Factor II = .26, Factor I versus Factor III = .14, and Factor II versus Factor III = .52. The within-instrument correlations found in the present study are shown in Part A of Table 4.2.

In the present study the correlations at the different rating occasions between Peterson Factors I and II varied between .38 and .52, considerably larger than the r value reported by Peterson. The Schaefer Factor I versus II correlations (.20 to .27) and the Schaefer Factor I versus III correlations (.12 to .18) were remarkably similar to those found by Schaefer and Aaronson; the Schaefer Factor II versus III correlations (.54 to .64) were slightly higher than the r value reported by Schaefer and Aaronson.

Cross-instrument correlations. Cross-instrument correlations appear in Part B of Table 4.2. It will be noted that the correlations of the corresponding factors from the two

Table 4.2 Psychometric Characteristics of Elementary School Instruments at the Four Rating Occasions

Factors	Grade			
	1st $N = 773$	2nd $N = 854$	3rd $N = 677$	4th $N = 323$
Part A: Within-instrument correlations				
Peterson Factor I vs. Peterson Factor II	.38	.44	.47	.52
Schaefer Factor I vs. Schaefer Factor II	.20	.25	.27	.21
Schaefer Factor I vs. Schaefer Factor III	.12	.14	.14	.18
Schaefer Factor II vs. Schaefer Factor III	.54	.64	.64	.62
Part B: Cross-instrument correlations				
Corresponding factors Peterson Factor I vs. Schaefer Factor I	−.62	−.64	−.65	−.57
Peterson Factor II vs. Schaefer Factor II	−.72	−.75	−.76	−.76
Non-corresponding factors Peterson Factor I vs. Schaefer Factor II	−.36	−.37	−.40	−.38
Peterson Factor II vs. Schaefer Factor I	−.07	−.11	−.10	−.11
Factor III Peterson Factor I vs. Schaefer Factor III	−.32	−.34	−.40	−.43
Peterson Factor II vs. Schaefer Factor III	−.74	−.75	−.78	−.74
Part C: Pooled instrument correlations				
Pooled Factor I vs. Pooled Factor II	.32	.36	.37	.38
Pooled Factor I vs. Schaefer Factor III	.26	.28	.30	.36
Pooled Factor II vs. Schaefer Factor III	.70	.75	.78	.75

Note.—On the Peterson instrument and pooled instrument scores, high scores = disturbance; on the Schaefer instrument, high scores = health.

instruments ranged from $-.57$ to $-.76$ over the four rating occasions; the median r was $-.69$, indicating congruence. The correlations between Peterson Factor II and Schaefer Factor I were small, ranging between $-.07$ and $-.11$, indicating independence; however, the correlations between Peterson Factor I and Schaefer Factor II were somewhat higher than desirable, running between $-.36$ and $-.40$.[9] This suggests that Peterson Factor I is not as pure a Factor I measure as desirable; it undoubtedly contains some contaminating Factor II items.

Because of the low correlation between Schaefer Factors III and I and the moderate correlation between Schaefer Factors III and II, we expected a similar pattern of relationships between Schaefer Factor III and the two Peterson dimensions. As may be seen in Part B of Table 4.2, the correlations between Peterson Factor I and Schaefer Factor III varied from $-.32$ to $-.43$ over the four rating occasions and were similar in magnitude to Peterson I versus Schaefer II; the correlations between Peterson Factor II and Schaefer Factor III ranged from $-.74$ to $-.78$ and were close in magnitude to Peterson II versus Schaefer II. Thus, although the Peterson Factor I versus Schaefer Factor III correlations were higher than desirable, they were considerably lower than the Peterson Factor II versus Schaefer Factor III correlations.

Pooling of elementary school instrument scores. In view of the congruence of the corresponding factor dimensions of the two instruments and in order to improve the reliability of the measurements, we pooled the Factor I scores from the two instruments, and we pooled the Factor II scores from the two instruments. Prior to pooling, the teachers' raw scores were converted to standard scores. In converting the scores from the Peterson and Schaefer instruments to standard scores, the first grade scores of all subjects were used as the standardization base; this procedure permitted us to use first grade as a base line against which age trends could be measured.

---

[9] Similar findings based on $N = 271$ were presented in the previous chapter (see Table 3.4).

Since the instruments have scores running in opposite directions (high Problem Checklist scores indicate disturbance; high Classroom Behavior Inventory scores indicate health), the signs of the scores from the latter instrument were reversed. High pooled instrument scores, therefore, represented emotional impairment. The rest of the procedure was identical to that described for the pooling of preschool instrument scores.

The correlations among the pooled factor scores are shown in Part C of Table 4.2. It may be seen that the correlations between the pooled Factors I and II and between pooled Factor I and Schaefer Factor III were relatively modest; however, not unexpectedly, *r* values between pooled Factor II and Schaefer Factor III were substantial.

Averaging across rating occasions. For the purpose of securing maximally stable measures for the longitudinal predictions, the pooled instrument scores, the scores on Global Impairment, and the scores on Referral were each averaged across various grade levels for certain specific data analyses. The number of grade levels averaged depended on the particular hypothesis tested. This will be explained further in later chapters.

Academic attainment

At each rating occasion during the preschool period, the teachers assessed the children on Verbal Fluency. The ratings of the two full-time teachers were pooled and to obtain maximally stable measures, the pooled scores were averaged over the preschool rating occasions.

In elementary school the data on the youngsters' achievement level were collected annually toward the end of each school year. The scores on the city-wide tests were obtained from the New York City Board of Education, as follows:

The Metropolitan School Readiness Test was administered one month after the first group of children (Cohort A) had entered first grade. Since the Board of Education subsequently discontinued this Test, these data were not available for Cohorts B and C.

The Verbal subtests of the Metropolitan Achievement Tests (Word Knowledge and Reading) were administered beginning with grade 2. Scores were obtained up to grade 4 for Cohort A children, through grade 3 for Cohort B children, and for grade 2 for Cohort C children. In order to secure maximally stable measures, the scores from the two subtests were pooled within each grade level.

The Arithmetic subtests of the Metropolitan Achievement Tests (Mathematics Concepts, Mathematics Problem Solving, and Mathematics Computation) were given to Cohorts A and B while they were in third grade (Cohort C had not reached the third grade by the end of the study). To maximize the stability of the Arithmetic achievement measure, the scores from the three subtests were averaged.

The children took these exams in groups in their classroom. A member of the research staff administered the same tests on an individual basis to the youngsters attending parochial or private schools.

The elementary school classroom teacher completed forms covering the other measures of academic attainment, i.e., Academic Standing and Verbal Fluency (beginning with first grade), Grade Placement (beginning with second grade), and Level Within Grade (on the last rating occasion when Cohorts A, B, and C were in fourth, third, and second grade, respectively).

Sample Attrition

In any prolonged longitudinal study with a large number of subjects, the problem of sample attrition must be given serious consideration. In the present study we made every effort within our means to keep track of our subjects and to locate missing subjects. While the children were still in day care, we kept in touch with the center directors to find out in which elementary school the children would be enrolling, and once the children had entered elementary school, we devised a number of different procedures to keep track of them.

In order to locate missing children, we consulted personnel in the last school which the child had attended, and we frequently made personal visits to the schools. Where those efforts failed,

Table 4.3 Percentage of Subjects on Whom Data Were Obtained

Sex and grade level	Expected *N*	% subjects with social-emotional data	% subjects with achievement data
Boys			
1st grade	628	62%	—
2nd grade	628	70%	64%
3rd grade	462	74%	66%
4th grade	216	74%	66%
Girls			
1st grade	602	62%	––
2nd grade	602	69%	66%
3rd grade	432	76%	68%
4th grade	209	79%	73%

we circulated missing children's lists throughout the entire New York City public and parochial school systems. The families often have long-term relationships with the day care centers and sometimes, when a child could not be located, we again contacted the day care center he had attended. On some occasions we paid visits to the families. Had we had more resources, we would have been able to get in touch with more families and decreased attrition even further.

While the children were in day care, sample attrition was moderate and non-selective with regard to the children's background (see Kohn & Rosman, 1972b). After the children had entered elementary school, attrition became a more serious problem. After the first year of the study we instituted a procedure which enabled us to keep track of the magnitude as well as any selectivity of attrition. At each point in data collection the major variables were coded twice: first, the actual score obtained by the subject, and second, whether or not the data were available on that variable for that subject. A subject was given a score of 1 if the information was obtained ("in") and a score of 0 if the datum was missing ("out"). We called this the missing data code.

Size of attrition

Table 4.3 shows the total number of subjects, separately for boys and girls, on whom data would have been collected had there been no sample attrition and the percentage of this total on whom we actually obtained data. The decreasing number of expected subjects from second grade level on is due to the fact that during the first and second grades, data could be collected on all three Cohorts, during the third grade only on Cohorts A and B, and in fourth grade only on the oldest group, Cohort A.

It may be seen that social-emotional data were obtained on 62% of all subjects in first grade and on 74% of the boys and 79% of the girls in fourth grade. It is noteworthy that the percentage of children on whom data were collected actually increased between the first and fourth grades. This is largely a reflection of the fact that, as the study progressed, we became more adept at locating missing subjects. All in all, we felt that to obtain a 74%–79% return during the fifth year of data collection in a study in which we relied primarily on mail contact with the schools was highly encouraging for future large-scale longitudinal and screening studies.

The percentage of children on whom we obtained achievement data (i.e., Word Knowledge and Reading test scores) was lower than the percentage of youngsters on whom we collected emotional impairment data. This was, in part, due to the fact that the availability of achievement scores was less affected by the efforts of the research staff. The public school testing program was always carried out on specific days during the school year, and if a child was absent on any of those days, he was not tested.

Selectivity of attrition

The loss of subjects raised the question of whether the children for whom we had data could be considered a random sample of the original group. By correlating the missing data codes with other variables, we were able to make definitive statements about the nature of the attrition. Two issues were examined: (a) whether subjects who had dropped out of the

Table 4.4 Extent to which Data Were Missed as a Function of Subjects' Preschool Emotional Impairment

Preschool syndrome measures	Social-emotional data				Achievement data		
	Grade				Grade		
	1st	2nd	3rd	4th	2nd	3rd	4th
				Part A: Boys			
	$N = 628$	628	462	216	$N = 628$	462	216
Apathy-Withdrawal Rating 1	−.07	−.08	.03	−.15*	−.10	.00	−.09
Anger-Defiance Rating 1	−.05	−.07	−.00	−.02	−.12**	−.03	−.03
				Part B: Girls			
	$N = 602$	602	432	209	$N = 602$	432	209
Apathy-Withdrawal Rating 1	−.03	.00	.03	−.05	−.06	−.01	−.05
Anger-Defiance Rating 1	−.09*	−.01	−.16**	−.17*	−.06	−.12**	−.19**

Note. — Obtained data were coded 1; missing data were coded 0.
For Apathy-Withdrawal and Anger-Defiance, high scores = disturbance.
*p ≤ .05.
**p ≤ .01.

sample were more severely disturbed, as measured on the first rating occasion (Rating 1), than subjects who were retained in the sample, and (b) whether the missing subjects differed from the remaining subjects on the demographic variables.

Attrition and emotional impairment at onset of study. The correlations between social-emotional and achievement "in" versus "out" data and the children's emotional impairment at Rating 1 are presented in Table 4.4, separately by sex. For the boys, there was no consistent pattern; 2 of 14 correlations were significant, suggesting that boys on whom fourth grade social-emotional data were collected were significantly lower on Apathy-Withdrawal than the missing subjects, and boys on whom second grade achievement scores were obtained were significantly lower on Anger-Defiance than the missing subjects. In other words, in both instances, boys who were more disturbed at the beginning of the research were lost from the study.

For the girls, there was a more consistent trend: None of the correlations between the "in" versus "out" data and Apathy-Withdrawal at Rating 1 were statistically significant but 5 of 7 correlations between "in" versus "out" data and Anger-Defiance at Rating 1 were. These results suggest that the girls who remained in the sample during the elementary school period were significantly lower on Anger-Defiance than the missing subjects. Again, it was the more disturbed children who were lost from the sample.

In sum, although the correlations were not large, we detected a tendency for the more disturbed children to drop out of the project.

Attrition and demographic variables. The social-emotional and achievement "in" versus "out" data were correlated with ten demographic variables; the findings appear in Table 4.5, separately for males and females. There is little evidence of selectivity of attrition among boys: Of 70 correlations, only 7 were significant at the 5% level or better; this could easily be a chance result.

For girls, there is some evidence of selectivity: 25 of 70 correlations were significant at the 5% level or better; these ranged from .09 to .19, with the median value a relatively low *r*

Table 4.5 Extent to which Data Were Missed as a Function of Subjects' Demographic Status

Demographic variables	Social-emotional data				Achievement data		
	Grade				Grade		
	1st	2nd	3rd	4th	2nd	3rd	4th
Part A: Boys							
	N = 617	617	453	212	*N* = 617	453	212
Age at Rating 1	.07	−.03	.03	.01	.01	.08	.01
Number of siblings	.10*	.05	.06	.01	.07	.02	−.01
Family intactness	−.12*	−.02	−.03	−.11	−.05	−.04	−.15*
White vs. Others	−.08	−.05	−.12**	−.08	−.06	−.08	−.13
Black vs. Puerto Rican	.06	.03	.04	−.04	.03	−.01	−.05
Social class	−.03	−.03	−.02	−.13	−.01	−.11*	−.11
Occupational level	.05	.04	.04	.11	.04	.03	.14*
Family income	.14**	09*	.04	.02	.13*	.09	.05
Welfare vs. other	.02	.00	−.00	.02	.03	.01	.04
Family stability	−.02	−.03	−.03	−.00	−.01	.04	.05
Part B: Girls							
	N = 593	593	425	206	*N* = 593	425	206
Age at Rating 1	.09*	.01	−.01	.01	.09*	.01	−.06
Number of siblings	.09*	.06	.12**	.15*	.04	.13**	.19**
Family intactness	−.05	−.08	−.04	−.12	−.11*	−.04	.19**
White vs. Others	−.07	−.13**	−.10*	−.14*	−.13**	−.05	−.11
Black vs. Puerto Rican	.06	.16**	.13**	−.02	.16**	.08	.01
Social class	−.01	.04	−.09	−.15*	.06	−.10*	−.12
Occupational level	.06	.12**	.09	.16*	.08	.14**	.17*
Family income	.08	.05	.01	.08	.13**	.05	.11
Welfare vs. other	.08	.06	−.06	−.05	.07	.01	−.01
Family stability	.03	.07	.02	.14*	.12**	−.01	.15*

Note.—Obtained data were coded 1; missing data were coded 0.

Demographic variables were scored as follows: family intactness: 1 = both parents at home, 2 = broken home; white vs. others: 1 = white, −1 = black or Puerto Rican; black vs. Puerto Rican: 1 = black, 0 = white; −1 = Puerto Rican; for social class and family income, high scores = highest levels; for occupational level, low scores = professional level; welfare vs. other: −1 = welfare, 0 = other assistance, 1 = self-supporting; family stability: from 1 = unstable to 5 = relatively stable.

*p ≤ .05.

**p ≤ .01.

= .13. In spite of the small size of the correlations, however, certain trends emerge. The bulk of the data suggests that, compared to the missing subjects, the girls retained in the sample came from more underprivileged backgrounds; i.e., families were larger, mothers tended to be more poorly educated, and the head of the household had a lower occupational level. Also, a larger number of black and Puerto Rican than white girls remained in the study. On the other hand, two variables point in the opposite direction: The families of girls on whom we continued to obtain data had somewhat higher incomes and were rated by the day care counselor to be more stable than the families of girls who were lost from the study. These contrary findings are difficult to interpret.

On balance, the data imply that the female subjects who remained in the study were socially more disadvantaged than the portion of the sample who dropped out of the project.

Male-female differences. Looking at both social-emotional and demographic data, we may conclude that boys showed only a slight amount of selectivity of attrition whereas the evidence pointed to some differences between the missing and remaining girls: Those who were retained in the sample tended to be less impaired on the Anger-Defiance syndrome and socially more deprived than girls who were lost from the study.

Why the difference in attrition between boys and girls? A comparison of the correlation matrices of the males with the correlation matrices of the females shows that hardly any of the correlations ran in opposite directions; the boys' data showed the same trends as the girls' but the effects were not as strong. In other words, the difference was one of degree and not of kind.

In conclusion, it should be noted that the correlation coefficients were generally low; the highest significant r value was .19, and the median of the significant correlations was $r = .13$. Thus, sample attrition introduced a very small bias, one which was not likely to influence unduly the results of the present study.

CHAPTER 5

Validity of Apathy-Withdrawal and Anger-Defiance as Measures of Emotional Impairment

Before we could proceed with the longitudinal study, we had to demonstrate the clinical relevance of the factor dimensions of the Symptom Checklist and the Social Competence Scale. We formulated two major hypotheses:

1. Children with known psychiatric disorders will score significantly higher on Apathy-Withdrawal and Anger-Defiance than a group of "normal" children.

2. Within the group of normal children, those judged to be more disturbed will score higher on Apathy-Withdrawal and Anger-Defiance than those judged to be less disturbed. More

specific hypotheses regarding the relative position of subgroups within the normal sample will be spelled out presently.

By "normal" children we meant the randomly selected day care sample. In any randomly selected group there will be a distribution ranging from healthy to disturbed; therefore, in speaking of a normal group, we were not implying that all the youngsters were healthy.

To test the first hypothesis, data collected on the first rating occasion in November 1967 (Rating 1) were compared with data from two independent reference groups of severely disturbed youngsters—namely, (a) children enrolled in three therapeutic day nurseries, and (b) children placed in a local mental hospital.[10]

To test the second hypothesis, data collected at Rating 1 were used to divide the longitudinal study sample into a series of reference groups of varying degrees of health and disturbance.

Validity studies are fraught with difficulties. Ideally, one would want the raters to be unaware of all contaminating information, such as a child's diagnostic status, level of pathology, and whether he was attending a regular community program, enrolled in a special school, or confined to an institution. In reality, this is hard to do. For example, in the present study the children in the therapeutic nurseries and mental hospital were rated by personnel at these facilities. There was a potential risk that the children in these groups would score high on Apathy-Withdrawal and Anger-Defiance simply because of the raters' knowledge that the youngsters had been placed into a special setting for disturbed children. Because of

---

[10]Originally, a third independent reference group nominated by the directors of the day care centers was studied but the group was dropped from the analysis because of lack of validity of the nominations. Inquiry revealed that the day care center directors had based their judgments on formal and informal reports by teachers, episodic observations of children in the classroom or in the hall, unsystematic parental reports, etc. The diversity of the sources and the unsystematic sampling of the sources were probably responsible for the lack of validity. For further details, see Kohn and Rosman (1973c).

limitations such as these, validity is best approached from a number of different angles. Therefore, we also used the teachers' global ratings (Global Impairment and Referral) to test the validity of the two syndrome measures, as will be shown in chapters 6 and 7.

Let us turn now to the subjects, methods, and results of the validity study.

Subjects

Independent reference groups

With the cooperation of three local therapeutic day nurseries and a local mental hospital (and with the consent of the parents), two samples of emotionally impaired children were selected. Since the youngsters had been placed in these facilities because of psychiatric disorders and upon the recommendation of a psychiatrist, we felt justified in assuming that the children in these groups would be more seriously disturbed than the random sample selected from the day care population.

1. *Therapeutic day nursery group:* All children age 7 or less enrolled in the three therapeutic day nurseries at the time of the study were included in the sample (N = 44; 31 boys, 13 girls). Of this group, 23 were judged to have severe emotional disturbance accompanied by mental retardation, 6 to be principally schizophrenic, and 15 to be autistic.

2. *Mental hospital group:* All children age 7 or less hospitalized at the time of the study were included in the sample (N = 30; 23 boys, 7 girls). Of this group, 5 were judged to have severe emotional disturbance accompanied by mental retardation, 19 were diagnosed as primarily schizophrenic and 5, as autistic (on one subject data were incomplete).

Reference groups in the day care sample

The longitudinal study sample was divided into five reference groups on the basis of the Global Impairment and Referral ratings made by the day care teachers at Rating 1. Separate reference groups were set up for boys (N = 628) and girls (N = 604), as follows:

1. *Well functioning group:* children who were rated by both day care teachers as well functioning and were not in treatment or in need of treatment (N = 175 boys, 244 girls);

2. *Moderately-well functioning group:* children who were rated by both teachers as moderately-well functioning or by one teacher as moderately-well functioning and by the other as well functioning and who were not in treatment or in need of treatment (N = 288 boys, 237 girls);

3. *Poorly functioning group:* children who were rated by both day care teachers as poorly functioning or by one teacher as poorly functioning and by the other as moderately-well functioning and who were not in treatment or in need of treatment (N = 39 boys, 32 girls);

4. *Remedial treatment group:* children receiving remedial treatment (e.g., for speech disorder) or requiring such help in the opinion of the head teacher (N = 52 boys, 45 girls);

5. *Therapy group:* children receiving psychiatric or psychological treatment or requiring such assistance in the opinion of the head teacher (N = 74 boys, 46 girls).

The first two groups may be considered emotionally healthy although we expected the Well functioning group to be, on average, healthier than the Moderately-well functioning group. The other three groups may be deemed disturbed since at least one teacher perceived the youngster to be coping inadequately or to need special help. By these criteria of disturbance, 26.3% of the boys and 20.3% of the girls in the day care sample were disturbed.

Hypothesized differences among reference groups. We developed three hypotheses regarding the relative standing of the various groups in the day care sample:

1. The children in the three disturbed groups (Poorly functioning, Remedial treatment, and Therapy) will have higher scores on Apathy-Withdrawal and Anger-Defiance than the two healthy groups (Well functioning and Moderately-well functioning).

2. Pathology will increase as we move from the Well functioning to the Moderately-well functioning to the disturbed groups.

3. Of the three disturbed groups, the Therapy group will have higher scores on the syndromes than the Poorly functioning and Remedial treatment groups. We felt that when youngsters are perceived as candidates for referral, they probably present a more serious problem in the classroom than children who are seen "merely" as coping poorly. Moreover, since previous research has shown a large discrepancy between number of children identified as disturbed and number receiving treatment (Kohn, 1968), we expected that only the most severely impaired youngsters would be in the Therapy group.

We were not sure of the relative position of the Remedial treatment group. These children generally have a specific and circumscribed problem (e.g., speech disorder), and we did not know to what extent this type of difficulty was symptomatic of more pervasive social-emotional impairment.

It should be noted that the comparison of the day care sample with the independent reference groups enabled us to draw more definitive conclusions about the validity of Apathy-Withdrawal and Anger-Defiance than the comparison among the reference groups within the day care sample since the criterion ratings of Global Impairment and Referral were made by the same teachers who assessed the children on the syndrome measures.

Methodology

Dependent variables

The dependent variables were the Apathy-Withdrawal and Anger-Defiance scores on the Symptom Checklist and the Social Competence Scale. These instruments were completed routinely by the day care teachers as part of the longitudinal study, and the teachers of the children in the independent reference groups used the same instruments. The Mental hospital group was also assessed by ward personnel; the teacher and ward personnel ratings were pooled and adjusted for the number of raters.

Demographic data

The same background information collected by the counselors attached to the day care centers (see chapter 4) was obtained

Table 5.1 Selected Demographic Variables for Day Care Sample and Independent Reference Groups

Demographic variables	Day care sample		Independent reference groups	
	All subjects $N = 1,232$	Disturbed groups $N = 288$	Therapeutic day nursery group $N = 44$	Mental hospital group $N = 29$
Mean age at rating (months)	54	54	75	68
Standard deviation of age	9.3	9.3	12.2	7.5
% male	51.0	56.7	70.5	76.7
% intact family	49.6	44.3	88.4	65.6
% race-ethnicity White Black Puerto Rican Other	27.0 55.8 15.6 1.5	28.7 52.8 16.4 2.1	82.9 17.1 00.0 00.0	63.0 25.9 11.1 00.0
Social class[a]	12	12	12	11
Median income ($)	5,300	5,000	8,000+	6,300

[a] Mean mother's education (years)
Adapted from Kohn and Rosman (1973c), p. 37.

for the children in the independent reference groups. To determine the comparibility of the day care sample and the independent reference groups, the means of the demographic variables were computed. The results are presented in Table 5.1 for the following groups: (a) entire day care sample, (b) disturbed children in the day care sample, (c) Therapeutic day nursery group, and (d) Mental hospital group.

It may be seen that the disturbed children in the day care sample were similar to the entire day care sample in all respects except sex and intactness of family: The disturbed groups in day care contained a considerably larger percentage of boys and a substantially smaller percentage of children from intact families. It is noteworthy that the day care disturbed children did not differ from the whole normative sample with respect to the percentage of children (a) from minority groups (black and Puerto Rican), and (b) from lower-class backgrounds.

Compared to the day care groups, the children in the independent reference groups were older; a higher percentage came from intact homes; there were more white and fewer black and Puerto Rican youngsters; and median family income was higher. The differences very likely reflect the selective factors which determine who receives therapeutic attention: Children from white, higher income, and intact families seem to have a better chance of getting into a treatment facility.

Correlations of demographic and dependent variables

To make sure that a comparison between the day care sample and the independent reference groups was not invalidated by these background differences, correlations between demographic data and the syndrome measures were calculated for the day care sample. The correlations appear in Table 5.2.

It is evident that the demographic variables accounted for only a samll amount of the variance of Apathy-Withdrawal and Anger-Defiance. There were a few significant differences— namely, (a) older children scored significantly lower (i.e., were less disturbed) than younger children on Apathy-Withdrawal; (b) boys scored significantly higher (i.e., were more disturbed) than girls on Anger-Defiance; (c) children from broken homes scored significantly higher on Anger-Defiance than children from intact families; and (d) children from lower-class backgrounds scored significantly higher on Apathy-Withdrawal than children from families higher on the social scale.

However, the correlations were generally small. The largest r (−.18) occurred between sex and Anger-Defiance, and we decided that the size of the coefficient warranted analyzing the data separately by sex. Since the other correlations were $r = .11$ or lower, it appeared unlikely that, after the groups had been separated by sex, differences in the remaining demographic data

Table 5.2 Correlations between Demographic Variables and Apathy-Withdrawal and Anger-Defiance Scores for the Day Care Sample

Demographic variables	Apathy-Withdrawal	Anger-Defiance
Age at rating	−0.06*	0.01
Sex	−0.06*	−0.18****
Family intactness	−0.04	0.11****
Race-ethnicity		
White versus Others	−0.01	0.02
Black versus Others	−0.01	0.03
Puerto Rican versus Others	0.00	0.01
Social class	−0.07*	0.02

Note.−*N* = 1,232.

Demographic variables were scored as follows: sex: 1 = male, 2 = female; family intactness: 1 = both parents at home, 2 = broken home; white versus others: 1 = white, 2 = others; black versus others: 1 = black, 2 = others; Puerto Rican versus others: 1 = Puerto Rican, 2 = others; for social class, high score = highest level.

For Apathy-Withdrawal and Anger-Defiance, high scores = disturbance.
    *$p \leqslant .05$.
****$p \leqslant .001$.
Adapted from Kohn and Rosman (1973c), p. 38.

could account for any appreciable differences among the reference group.[11]

Results

Comparison of day care sample with independent reference groups

The means and standard deviations of the Apathy-Withdrawal and Anger-Defiance scores are presented in Table 5.3, separately for boys and girls. Because the syndrome scores from each of the two preschool instruments were standardized, and scores from the two instruments were subsequently pooled (see chapter

[11] A detailed presentation of the relationship between demographic variables and measures of emotional impairment will be presented in chapter 7.

Table 5.3 Day Care, Therapeutic Day Nursery, and Mental Hospital Groups: Comparison of Syndrome Scores

Sex and groups	N	Means		Standard deviations	
		Apathy-Withdrawal	Anger-Defiance	Apathy-Withdrawal	Anger-Defiance
Boys					
Day care	628	0.12	0.33	1.83	1.99
Therapeutic day nursery	31	3.05***	2.53***	1.95	1.31
Mental hospital	23	2.08***	1.69***	1.82	1.70
Girls					
Day care	604	−0.12	−0.34	1.88	1.77
Therapeutic day nursery	13	2.90***	1.97***	1.99	1.58
Mental hospital	7	1.52*	2.62***	1.82	1.42

Note.−* and *** indicate that the mean differed significantly from the corresponding mean in the day care group at the .05 and .005 level, respectively.

The higher the score, the higher the level of pathology.

Adapted from Kohn and Rosman (1973c), p. 40.

4), the means of the Apathy-Withdrawal and Anger-Defiance scores of the children in the day care sample were close to 0 and the standard deviations, close to 2. Since a high score indicated disturbance, mean scores above 0 were in the direction of pathology, and mean scores below 0 were in the direction of health.

Boys as well as girls in the two independent reference groups scored significantly higher on both syndromes than the total day care sample; the average scores of the independent reference groups were 1 to 1½ standard deviations above the means of the normal children.[12]

[12] The tests of significance were carried out by means of the "Quick Test" (Cohen & Cohen, 1971), a rapid scoring but close approximation of the *t* test. In our calculations we used the standard deviation from the larger group and the *N* from the smaller group. This procedure produces a conservative estimate; comparisons which are of borderline significance may be significant when the exact *t* value is calculated.

Thus, the first major hypothesis, that children with known psychiatric disturbances would score significantly higher on Apathy-Withdrawal and Anger-Defiance than a group of normal children, was confirmed.

Comparison of five reference groups in day care

Table 5.4 shows the means and standard deviations of the syndrome scores of the reference groups in day care (as well as

Table 5.4 Five Reference Groups in the Day Care Sample and Two Independent Reference Groups: Comparison of Syndrome Scores

Groups	N	Means		Standard deviations	
		Apathy-Withdrawal	Anger-Defiance	Apathy-Withdrawal	Anger-Defiance
Part A: Boys					
Day care reference groups					
Healthy					
Well functioning	175	−1.41	−0.98	0.98	1.18
Moderately-well functioning	288	0.15	0.16	1.70	1.57
Disturbed					
Poorly functioning	39	2.17	2.04	1.48	2.27
Remedial treatment	52	1.22	1.52	2.39	2.06
Therapy	74	1.76	2.38	1.97	3.17
Independent reference groups					
Therapeutic day nursery	31	3.05	2.53	1.95	1.31
Mental hospital	23	2.08	1.69	1.82	1.70
Part B: Girls					
Day care reference groups					
Healthy					
Well functioning	244	−1.46	−1.05	0.93	1.23
Moderately-well functioning	237	0.28	−0.31	1.42	1.33
Disturbed					
Poorly functioning	32	2.05	0.58	1.97	1.82
Remedial treatment	45	1.24	0.47	2.03	2.23
Therapy	46	2.03	1.84	2.05	2.82
Independent reference groups					
Therapeutic day nursery	13	2.90	1.97	1.99	1.58
Mental hospital	7	1.52	2.62	1.82	1.42

Note.—Scores below 0 are in the direction of health; scores above 0 are in the direction of pathology.

Adapted from Kohn and Rosman (1973c), p. 40.

Table 5.5 Five Reference Groups in the Day Care Sample and Two Independent Reference Groups: Differences between Means and Their Statistical Significance

Girls	Boys						
	Well functioning	Moderately-well functioning	Poorly functioning	Remedial treatment	Therapy	Therapeutic day nursery	Mental hospital
Part A: Apathy-Withdrawal							
Day care reference groups							
Well functioning		−1.56***	−3.58***	−2.63***	−3.17***	−4.46***	−3.49***
Moderately-well functioning	−1.74***		−2.02***	−1.07***	−1.61***	−2.90***	−1.93***
Poorly functioning	−3.51***	−1.77***		0.95*	0.41	0.88**	0.09
Remedial treatment	−2.70***	−0.96***	0.81		0.54	−1.83***	−0.86
Therapy	−3.49***	−1.75***	0.02	−0.79*		−1.29**	−0.32
Independent reference groups							
Therapeutic day nursery	−4.36***	−2.62***	−0.85	−1.66*	−0.87		0.97*
Mental hospital	−2.98***	−1.24	0.53	−0.28	0.51	1.38	
Part B: Anger-Defiance							
Day care reference groups							
Well functioning		−1.14***	−3.02***	−2.50***	−3.36***	−3.51***	−2.67***
Moderately-well functioning	−0.74***		−1.88***	−1.36***	−2.22***	−2.37***	−1.53***
Poorly functioning	−1.63***	−0.74**		0.52	−0.34	−0.49	−0.35
Remedial treatment	−1.52***	−0.78***	0.11		−0.86	−1.01*	−0.17
Therapy	−2.89***	−2.15***	−1.26*	−1.37**		−0.15	0.69
Independent reference groups							
Therapeutic day nursery	−3.02***	−2.28***	−1.39*	−1.50	0.13		0.84*
Mental hospital	−3.67***	−2.93***	−2.04*	−2.15*	−0.78	−0.65	

Note.—In both parts of the table, values above the diagonal are comparisons among boys and values below the diagonal, comparisons among girls.

  *$p \leqslant .05$.
  **$p \leqslant .01$.
  ***$p \leqslant .005$.
  Adapted from Kohn and Rosman (1973c), p. 41.

the data of the independent reference groups), separately for boys and girls; the differences between the means and the statistical significance of the differences among the Apathy-Withdrawal scores and among the Anger-Defiance scores appear in Table 5.5, also separately by sex. The tests of significance were carried out by means of the "Quick Test" (see footnote 12).

The data support the second major assumption—namely, that in a group of normal children, the more disturbed youngsters would score higher on Apathy-Withdrawal and Anger-Defiance than the less disturbed children. Specifically, the following pattern is discernable with respect to the relative standing of the five reference groups in the day care sample:

1. In line with expectations, the Apathy-Withdrawal and Anger-Defiance scores of the three disturbed groups were significantly higher than the scores of the two healthy groups, both for boys and girls.

2. As anticipated, pathology increased as we proceeded from the Well functioning to the Moderately-well functioning to the disturbed groups. For both sexes: (a) The means of the Well functioning group were substantially below 0 on both syndromes; because of the curvilinear relationship between the Symptom Checklist and Social Competence Scale scores (see chapter 3), we can be certain that the children in the Well functioning group did not simply manifest a low level of symptoms but showed positive mental health. (b) The means of the Moderately-well functioning group were close to the average score of the entire day care sample—namely, 0. (c) The three disturbed groups all had scores well above 0, indicating emotional impairment.

3. The hypothesis regarding the rank order of the three disturbed groups was not confirmed at all for boys but was borne out partially for girls. Girls in the Therapy group scored significantly higher on Anger-Defiance than girls in the Poorly functioning and Remedial treatment groups; however, on Apathy-Withdrawal only the difference between the scores of the Therapy group and the Remedial treatment group reached significance. For both sexes, the Remedial treatment group had

the lowest pathology scores of the three disturbed day care groups.

Comparison of independent reference groups with day care reference groups

Difference among groups. We were interested in comparing the two independent reference groups with the subgroups in the day care sample. As may be seen in Table 5.4 and 5.5, on both syndromes, the strongest and most highly significant differences occurred between the scores of the independent reference groups and the two healthy day care groups. The pattern was true of boys and girls.

Of the seven groups in the study, the four most disturbed were the Poorly functioning and Therapy groups in day care and the Therapeutic day nursery and Mental hospital groups. Surprisingly, however, the scores of the independent reference groups were not consistently higher than the scores of the two day care groups. These four groups did not show the progression of successively higher means that we had expected.

Boys in the Therapeutic day nursery group scored significantly higher on Apathy-Withdrawal than boys in the Therapy group but on Anger-Defiance the differences between the scores were not significant nor were any differences between the scores of the Mental hospital group and those of the two most disturbed day care groups significant (see Table 5.5). For girls, there were small but significant differences between the independent reference groups and the Poorly functioning day care group on Anger-Defiance.

Sex differences. To obtain a clearer picture of sex differences in patterns of disturbance, we examined the difference between the Apathy-Withdrawal and Anger-Defiance scores for each of the groups. Some sex differences emerged. The boys in the three disturbed day care reference groups had high scores on both syndrome measures; the Apathy-Withdrawal and Anger-Defiance scores were approximately equal, and none of the differences (*t* test for correlated means) were significant. The pattern was the same for the independent reference groups.

All three day care groups of disturbed girls also had high scores on Apathy-Withdrawal but only the Therapy group had a high score on Anger-Defiance. The difference between the Apathy-Withdrawal and Anger-Defiance scores of the Poorly functioning and Remedial treatment groups were at a statistically significant level (t = 2.34, $p \leqslant .02$ and t = 2.00, $p \leqslant .05$, respectively) but there was no significant difference between the Therapy group's Apathy-Withdrawal and Anger-Defiance scores (t = .75, $p \leqslant .20$). The findings indicate that girls who showed predominantly Apathy-Withdrawal pathology were not considered candidates for referral whereas girls who manifested Anger-Defiance symptoms, alone or in combination with inhibited functioning, were likely to be referred for treatment of personality disturbance.

This line of reasoning is supported by the data from the two independent reference groups, each of whom scored high (means of 1.5 or above) on both syndromes. In other words, the evidence suggests that girls in treatment are not representative of all disturbed girls. If a girl exhibits both recessive and hostile behavior or only hostile behavior, her chances of receiving therapy are greater than if she is "merely" apathetic and withdrawn.

Comments

Two issues merit special attention: First, why the pathology scores did not increase in the expected direction. Since the Poorly functioning and Therapy groups in day care and the two independent reference groups all had mean scores in the general area of 2, our concern that rater awareness that the subjects were in a special setting for emotionally impaired children would result in higher scores on the syndromes was unfounded. On the contrary, we were faced with the question of why children who were so deviant that they could not be enrolled in a community facility did not differ more significantly from the two most disturbed day care groups.

Since it is plausible to assume that children attending a therapeutic day nursery or confined in a mental hospital have more severe disorders than disturbed children at day care centers, the absence of significant differences is probably a function of the frame of reference of the raters. The teachers in the therapeutic day nurseries and the mental hospital are in continuous contact with emotionally impaired children and may become so accustomed to deviant functioning that they do not rate it as severely as the day care teachers who also deal with many healthy youngsters. Another possible explanation is that our instruments were not sensitive to extreme forms of pathology and, therefore, an arbitrary limit was imposed on the severity of disturbance that could be recorded.

The second issue raised by the results was why the boys in the Poorly functioning group did not differ significantly from the boys in the Therapy group. (For girls, angry-defiant behavior was found to be one factor leading to referral.) We can only surmise that in the case of boys it is not solely emotional impairment as detected by the instruments which results in referral for therapeutic intervention. There must be other characteristics, undetected by the instruments, which, alone or in combination with the variables assessed by our scales, cause teachers to refer some boys and not to refer others who may be equally as disturbed. Our findings suggest that boys who are referred are among the most disturbed but we cannot say why some emotionally impaired boys are perceived as requiring treatment while others are not. In this respect our results differ from those of Shepherd et al. (1971) who asserted: "It appeared, then, that for the majority of children neither the clinical nor the statistical methods of assessing abnormality indicated that degree of disturbance was the main factor leading to referral for psychiatric treatment" (p. 136).

Conclusions

Although the analysis of the reference groups did not yield the expected gradation among the disturbed groups, the data nevertheless strongly suggest that the patterns of behavior detected by the Symptom Checklist and the Social Competence Scale were valid indicators of emotional impairment. The major evidence in support of this position is:

1. The two groups of children with known clinical disorders, i.e., the Therapeutic day nursery and Mental hospital groups,

scored significantly and substantially higher on Apathy-Withdrawal and Anger-Defiance than the entire day care sample.

2. The four most disturbed groups, i.e., the Poorly functioning and Therapy groups of the day care sample and the two independent reference groups, showed substantially higher levels of pathology than the two healthy groups of the day care sample, i.e., the Well functioning and Moderately-well functioning groups.

These conclusions with regard to validity are corroborated by the findings of Rutter et al. (1970) who asked teachers to complete an instrument which assessed two dimensions of behavior which the researchers labeled "neurotic" and "antisocial." As noted in chapter 2, neurotic behavior corresponded closely to the Apathy-Withdrawal syndrome of the present study, and antisocial behavior was conceptually similar to Anger-Defiance. Using the evaluation of male psychiatrists as their criterion of validity, the investigators found a high degree of agreement between the teachers' ratings and the independent psychiatric assessments with respect to (a) level of disturbance, and (b) type of disturbance; most of the children who were categorized as neurotic on the basis of the teacher questionnaire were similarly identified by the psychiatrists, and the same was true of the youngsters who were considered antisocial.

CHAPTER 6

Social-Emotional Functioning and Academic Attainment: Sex and Age Differences

We now turn to the findings of the longitudinal study. For each major topic in this and subsequent chapters, we will present a brief review of the relevant literature, a statement of our hypotheses, a report of the results, and some observations on our findings.

In this chapter we will focus on social-emotional functioning and academic attainment as related to sex and age variables.

SOCIAL-EMOTIONAL FUNCTIONING

It will be recalled that the social-emotional variables for the preschool period were Apathy-Withdrawal, Anger-Defiance,

Global Impairment, and Referral. The same variables were measured during the elementary school period, with the addition of one other, Low Task Orientation.

Sex Differences

There is substantial evidence that, during the elementary school years, emotional impairment is more widespread among boys than among girls. Most of the investigators who have studied samples of normal children have found a larger number of boys exhibiting serious maladjustment than girls. For example, Wickman (1928) reported that 10% of boys as compared to 3% of girls were considered to have severe behavior problems. In the Rogers (1942) study, the percentages were 18% for boys and 7% for girls and in Ullman's (1952) investigation, 13% and 3%, respectively. Similar results were also obtained by Bower (1969), Cummings (1944), and Olson (1930).

In the bulk of these studies, two kinds of measures were used: (a) global ratings of maladjustment (see Bower, 1969; Ullman, 1952; among others), and/or (b) a series of behavior ratings or indices, relevant to the adjustment-maladjustment continuum, which were summed and treated as if they measured a single fundamental dimension of emotional impairment (see Olson, 1930; Rogers, 1942; Ullman, 1952).

When, instead of applying global or other one-dimensional measures of disturbance, investigators looked at specific symptoms of deviant functioning, they generally observed that acting-out behavior was more prevalent among boys than girls; symptoms such as passivity, shyness, and anxiety were found to occur either as often in boys as girls or somewhat more frequently in girls.

For example, Macfarlane et al. (1954) stated: "Boys are more likely to have the following problems: *overactivity, attention demanding, jealousy, competitiveness, lying, selfishness in sharing, temper tantrums,* and *stealing.* The girls, on the other hand, are more likely than boys to *suck their thumbs,* be *excessively modest* and *reserved, fuss about their food,* be *timid, shy, fearful, oversensitive, somber,* and have *mood swings*" (p. 156). Cullen and Boundy (1966b) also reported that boys were higher on destructiveness and disorders associated with social standards while girls were higher on lethargy, thumbsucking, etc. (see also Lapouse & Monk, 1964; Mensh, Kantor, Domke, Gildea, & Glidewell, 1959; Ryle, Pond, & Hamilton, 1965; von Harnack, 1953).

Researchers examining total populations obtained results consistent with those found in samples of normal children. In Bremer's (1951) study of all 5- to 14-year-olds living on an island off the coast of Norway, 17.2% of boys as compared to 7.9% of girls manifested the aggressive syndrome pattern, and 14.3% of girls as compared to 11.7% of boys showed evidence of what he called the "aesthenic" symptom cluster (passivity, repression, fear).

Rutter et al. (1970), who studied all 10- and 11-year-old youngsters with homes on the Isle of Wight, noted a substantially higher prevalence of "antisocial" (read angry-defi-ant) behavior among boys than girls while a slightly lower proportion of boys than girls showed "neurotic" (i.e., apathetic-withdrawn) disorders.[13]

Although the categories of behavior traits used by Bremer and Rutter et al. are similar to the syndrome measures of Apathy-Withdrawal and Anger-Defiance employed in the present study, these investigators made the assumption that the symptom patterns were mutually exclusive. In fact, as we have shown, the dimensions are relatively uncorrelated and, therefore, co-exist: An individual can score high on both syndromes or can score low on both syndromes or can score high on one and low on the other.

Hypotheses

We formulated the following hypotheses:

---

[13] It is interesting to note that these sex differences seem to hold throughout the human life span, at least in western culture. In their review of the literature of epidemiological studies of psychiatric disorders in adults, Dohrenwend and Dohrenwend (1969) found that men exhibited psychopathy, i.e., acting-out disorders, in larger number than women while women tended to show evidence of "neurotic" disorders more than men did.

1. With respect to *differences between the sexes*, we expected that (a) boys would show more acting-out behavior and, therefore, would receive higher scores on Anger-Defiance and Low Task Orientation than girls; we anticipated slight, if any, sex differences on Apathy-Withdrawal; and (b) boys would receive higher scores than girls on Global Impairment and Referral.

2. Regarding *within-sex differences*, we predicted that boys would be significantly more disturbed on Anger-Defiance and Low Task Orientation than on Apathy-Withdrawal; conversely, girls would show more impairment on Apathy-Withdrawal than on the other two syndromes.

Age Differences

Age differences, like sex differences, have been assessed with different measures (global ratings, one-dimensional aggregates, specific symptoms, and constellations of symptoms, i.e., syndromes).

In a number of epidemiological studies, the approach has been to determine the extent to which the prevalence of specific symptoms changes with age. Investigators examining behavior traits indicative of deviant functioning found that some increased with age, some decreased, and others remained relatively stable over time. For example, Cummings (1944) in her study of 2- to 7-year-old children observed a significant decrease in difficulties in bladder control and specific fears (animals, loud noises) between the ages of 2 and 7 but an increase in lack of concentration and daydreaming during the same period. Other symptoms, such as restlessness and symptoms of general anxiety, showed no consistent age trends.

Similarly, Macfarlane et al.'s longitudinal study of children aged 21 months to 14 years revealed a decline in speech difficulties and problems related to biological control (soiling and enuresis) and to the "energetic expression" of aggression (destructiveness, temper tantrums, overactivity) as the children grew older. The changes in the symptoms suggest the importance of maturation and training (see also Ackerson, 1931, 1942; Lapouse & Monk, 1958, 1964; Shepherd et al., 1971).

Another approach has been to measure average number of symptoms per child. Lapouse and Monk reported that symptoms of disturbed functioning reached a peak during the preschool period and subsequently leveled off. Cullen and Boundy found that the average number of problems per child climbed until the 6- to 7-year range and then remained fairly stable until age 12 for boys and age 14 for girls. Cummings' sample of 2- to 7-year-olds showed no change in average number of symptoms at the various age levels. Macfarlane et al. also noted no age trends in incidence figures between 21 months and age 11; from ages 12 to 14 there was a decline in the average number of symptoms for both sexes (Macfarlane et al., 1954, p. 158). Olson found no change in problem tendencies in school-age children up to age 12 but noted an increase thereafter (13- to 15-year-olds).

One of the few researchers who has studied the extent to which syndromes of emotional impairment (in contrast to specific symptoms) vary with age is Peterson (1961) who found that both Personality problems and Conduct problems declined in severity between kindergarten and fourth grade but thereafter became more serious. Peterson speculated that the subsequent increase in severity might arise from the early agitation of adolescence; this would also account for the increase, in early adolescence, in the average number of symptoms per child reported by Olson.

It is clear that the research findings on age differences are less consistent from one study to another than the findings on sex differences. The variability in results may very likely be due to the fact that different investigators sampled different problems. For example, symptoms that recede with increasing maturation (such as enuresis and speech difficulties) will show a peak during the early years; on the other hand, behavior traits related to difficulties in attending to a structured task (such as daydreaming, restlessness, and boredom) may be more prevalent during the school years. Since incidence of specific problems and symptoms is a function of stage of development, maturational level, and social expectations, increases or decreases in average number of symptoms per child across wide age ranges may simply reflect the particular categories of symptoms tapped and their relevance to the age level of the children under study.

The lack of consensus suggests that age per se is not a variable—other things vary with age, e.g., the setting in which children function (home, school), the expectations of others (parents, teachers), biological and maturational changes, etc. In the present study we will examine age trends in school functioning; therefore, Rogers' (1942) study is of special interest because it suggests that environmental differences may account for some of the variations in level of impairment. Rogers combined a variety of criteria into a single aggregate measure of disturbance. He carried out his research in various schools; in some he found an increase in prevalence of emotional impairment between the ages of 6 and 13, in others a decrease over the same age span. Rogers speculated that the differences in level of pathology might be related to differences in school policies. For example, a school in which an increase in disturbance was found did not have special ability groupings; thus, the brighter students were forced to slow down while for the duller students the pace was too rapid.

There are two theoretical positions on the influence of the environment which have a bearing on the relationship between age and social-emotional functioning. According to "crisis theorists," such as Lindeman (1944) and Caplan (1955), entry into school represents a period of heightened stress leading to an initial increase in disturbance; this is followed later by a drop in the level of pathology as most children make a more-or-less successful adaptation to life at school.

In recent years the non-educational aspects of the school experience have gained increasing recognition. Barbara Biber and her associates (Biber, 1961; Biber, Gilkeson, & Winsor, 1959; Minuchin, Biber, Shapiro, & Zimiles, 1969) have been vigorous champions of the position that, as a socializing institution, the school is second in importance only to the family and can have considerable impact on the child's mental health, either for better or for worse. Decreasing or increasing levels of disturbance can be taken as indicative of the extent to which the school is exerting a wholesome or detrimental influence on the youngsters' social-emotional functioning.

The data of the present study were examined in the light of these two theoretical formulations; however, no specific hypotheses were developed.

Results

Apathy-Withdrawal, Anger-Defiance, and Low Task Orientation

The scores on the syndromes of emotional impairment are presented in Table 6.1, separately for boys and girls. The level of significance of the sex differences can be found in the last column of the table.

Male-female differences. The data show that in preschool boys were significantly more impaired than girls not only on Anger-Defiance, as anticipated, but also on Apathy-Withdrawal; however, the difference between the sexes was considerably larger on the former syndrome than on the latter.

In elementary school boys were significantly more disturbed than girls on each of the three syndromes at almost every grade

Table 6.1 Apathy-Withdrawal, Anger-Defiance, and Low Task Orientation as a Function of Sex and Age

Syndrome measures	Boys			Girls			Sex diff.
	N	Mean	SD	N	Mean	SD	t value
Part A: Preschool							
Apathy-Withdrawal	628	2.72	165.15	602	−31.60	158.00	3.70****
Anger-Defiance	628	43.20	187.00	602	−29.33	169.63	7.05****
Part B: Elementary school							
Apathy-Withdrawal							
1st grade	396	8.08	92.70	383	−8.87	87.32	2.66***
2nd grade	439	18.59	94.76	417	−4.94	86.96	3.75****
3rd grade	343	22.37	89.59	327	8.89	93.02	1.89
4th grade	159	22.12	90.23	164	2.58	82.43	2.02*
Anger-Defiance							
1st grade	396	20.20	99.49	383	−20.74	81.23	6.26****
2nd grade	439	41.36	107.74	417	−17.35	92.63	8.49****
3rd grade	343	38.71	104.92	327	−10.21	89.86	6.44****
4th grade	159	36.31	103.68	164	−23.50	87.93	5.53****
Low Task Orientation							
1st grade	396	19.85	99.29	378	−20.79	96.58	5.71****
2nd grade	438	35.60	102.46	416	−12.33	92.38	7.12****
3rd grade	341	35.56	99.82	327	−14.79	90.75	6.76****
4th grade	159	31.31	93.31	164	−23.56	88.72	5.36****

Note.—Preschool scores were averaged over all preschool rating occasions. High scores indicate emotional impairment.

*p ⩽ .05.
**p ⩽ .02.
***p ⩽ .01.
****p ⩽ .001.

level.[14] All but one of the differences were statistically significant, and the differences on Anger-Defiance and Low Task Orientation appear enormous (*t* values range from 5.36 to 8.49). The hypothesis that boys would be more disturbed than girls on Anger-Defiance and Low Task Orientation was confirmed.

Contrary to expectation, boys were also significantly more impaired than girls on Apathy-Withdrawal although (a) the differences in the scores were considerably smaller than the differences between boys' and girls' Anger-Defiance and Low Task Orientation scores, and (b) sex differences were less substantial as the children grew older; they were nonsignificant in third grade and significant only at the .05 level in fourth grade.

Within-sex differences.[15] To analyze within-sex differences, each child's Apathy-Withdrawal score was subtracted from his or her Anger-Defiance and Low Task Orientation scores, and the differences were tested for significance. The results appear in Table 6.2.

During the preschool period and at every grade level in elementary school the boys were more impaired on the two acting-out syndromes of Anger-Defiance and Low Task Orientation than on Apathy-Withdrawal. All differences were in this direction, and seven of nine differences were statistically significant at the 5% level or better.

For the girls the trend was in the opposite direction: With the exception of the preschool period, when the difference between the mean scores was small, the girls had significantly higher scores on Apathy-Withdrawal than on the other two syndromes. Seven of nine differences were statistically significant at the 5% level or better.

The hypotheses regarding within-sex differences were fully confirmed.

[14] As stated in chapter 4, each child was kept with the age cohort to which he belonged; therefore, the terms, "age" and "grade," are equivalents and may be used interchangeably.
[15] It was possible to make these comparisons since all data were converted to standard scores with the Rating 1 scores as the standardization base for the preschool data and the grade 1 data as the standardization base for the elementary school data.

Table 6.2 Within-Sex Differences of Severity of Impairment on the Acting-Out Syndromes of Anger-Defiance and Low Task Orientation versus Apathy-Withdrawal

Syndrome measures	Boys		Girls	
	Mean diff.	*t* value	Mean diff.	*t* value
Preschool Anger-Defiance versus Apathy-Withdrawal	40.48	4.97****	2.27	.30
Elementary school Anger-Defiance versus Apathy-Withdrawal				
1st grade	12.13	2.15*	−11.87	−2.30**
2nd grade	22.77	3.99****	−12.41	−2.53**
3rd grade	16.33	2.83***	−19.10	−3.24***
4th grade	14.20	1.58	−26.08	−3.88****
Low Task Orientation versus Apathy-Withdrawal				
1st grade	11.77	2.03*	−12.16	−2.04*
2nd grade	17.55	3.03***	−7.62	−1.45
3rd grade	13.01	2.15*	−23.67	−3.89****
4th grade	9.18	1.05	−26.15	−3.62****

Note.—To obtain difference scores, the Apathy-Withdrawal scores were subtracted from the Anger-Defiance and Low Task Orientation scores.
   *$p \leqslant .05$.
   **$p \leqslant .02$.
   ***$p \leqslant .01$.
   ****$p \leqslant .001$.

The findings on between-sex and within-sex differences are illustrated in Figures 3 and 4. Figure 3 displays data for the four years of elementary school; Figure 4 represents Apathy-Withdrawal and Anger-Defiance scores from first grade (any other age level would have served as well for illustrative purposes).

Age differences. Since different instruments were used to assess preschool and elementary school Apathy-Withdrawal and Anger-Defiance (see chapter 4), it was not possible to compare preschool and elementary school results. Changes in scores from one grade to another in elementary school (as presented in Table

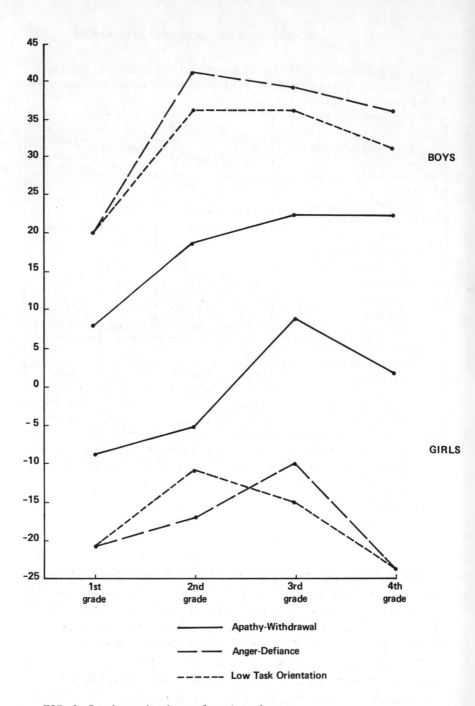

FIG. 3. Syndrome levels as a function of age.

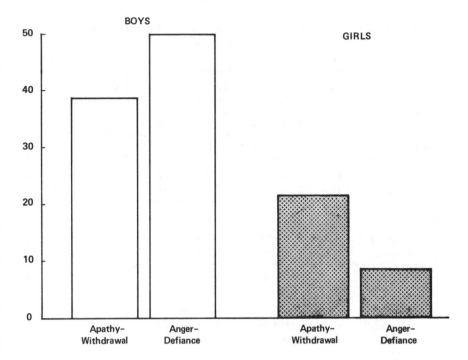

FIG. 4. Between-sex and within-sex differences on Apathy-Withdrawal and Anger-Defiance in first grade.

Note. In order to avoid negative scores, a constant of 30 was added to each of the four scores in this figure.

6.1 and Figure 3) were tested for significance;[16] these data appear in Table 6.3. We will examine age trends using each grade in turn as a base line against which to compare scores obtained

[16] In calculating the significance of differences between two age levels, we took advantage of the fact that the samples at each level consisted of two types of cases: (a) those who had a score at both age levels, and (b) those who had a score only at one age level. Using the former, we had the advantage of the correlated *t* test but with a smaller *N*; using the latter, we had the advantage of a larger *N* but we lost the information due to the correlation. The following formula allowed us to calculate the *t* value using both cases:

$$t = \frac{\overline{X}_1 - \overline{Y}_2}{\sqrt{(SE_{X_1})^2 = (SE_{Y_2})^2 - \dfrac{2 \text{ common cases} \times SD_{X_1} \times SD_{Y_2} \times r_{XY}}{N_X \times N_Y}}}$$

Table 6.3 Age Difference on Apathy-Withdrawal, Anger-Defiance, and Low Task Orientation

Sex and grade level	Mean diff.	*t* value 1st grade versus	Mean diff.	*t* value 2nd grade versus	Mean diff.	*t* value 3rd grade versus
Part A: Apathy-Withdrawal						
Boys						
2nd grade	10.51	2.06*				
3rd grade	14.29	2.43**	3.77	0.70		
4th grade	14.04	1.78	3.51	0.46	−0.26	0.04
Girls						
2nd grade	3.93	0.80				
3rd grade	17.76	3.19***	13.83	2.59***		
4th grade	11.46	1.63	7.52	1.06	−6.30	−0.92
Part B: Anger-Defiance						
Boys						
2nd grade	21.16	4.00****				
3rd grade	18.50	2.93***	−2.00	−0.45		
4th grade	16.11	1.89	−5.00	−0.57	−2.39	0.29
Girls						
2nd grade	3.39	0.72				
3rd grade	10.53	1.99*	7.14	1.37		
4th grade	−2.76	.38	−6.15	−0.90	−17.29	−2.54*
Part C: Low Task Orientation						
Boys						
2nd grade	15.84	2.94***				
3rd grade	15.71	2.45**	−0.14	−0.01		
4th grade	11.45	1.44	−4.39	−0.55	−4.26	−0.57
Girls						
2nd grade	8.46	1.66				
3rd grade	6.01	1.04	−2.45	−0.47		
4th grade	−2.78	.37	−11.24	−1.50	−8.78	−1.21

Note.—A difference in the positive direction indicates an increase in disturbance; a negative difference indicates a decline in disturbance.

*$p \leqslant .05$.
**$p \leqslant .02$.
***$p \leqslant .01$.
****$p \leqslant .001$.

at succeeding grades and thus assess the increase or decrease in the level of pathology.

On Apathy-Withdrawal, boys were significantly more impaired at the end of second and third grade than at the end of their first year in school; the difference between first and fourth grade scores approached significance ($p \leqslant .1$). After second grade, the increases in disturbance were too small to be significant.

The girls' Apathy-Withdrawal scores were significantly higher in third grade than they had been both in first and second grade. After third grade, no further significant change occurred.

On Anger-Defiance, the boys' sharp rise in impairment in second and third grade over the first grade level was highly significant, with the difference between first and fourth grade scores approaching significance ($p \leqslant .1$). The boys reached an asymptote in second grade, and no further significant changes occurred over the next two years.

In third grade the girls were significantly more disturbed on Anger-Defiance than in first grade. But the following year they improved significantly so that at the end of the fourth year of elementary school, the girls received approximately the same score on this syndrome as when they entered school.

On Low Task Orientation, the boys' level of functioning deteriorated significantly in second and third grade as compared to first grade. After second grade, the changes were not significant. The girls' scores fluctuated during the first four years of elementary school but none of the differences between grade levels was significant.

Global Impairment

Data on Global Impairment can be found in Table 6.4 and Figure 5, separately by sex. Since the same rating scales were used in day care and in elementary school, meaningful comparisons can be made among all rating occasions.

It will be recalled that Global Impairment was a 3-point scale whose points were defined as "well functioning" = 1, "moderately-well functioning" = 2, and "poorly functioning" = 3. As predicted, boys received higher scores than girls: The

Table 6.4 Global Impairment and Referral as a Function of Sex and Age

Global measures	Boys			Girls			Sex diff.
	N	Mean	SD	N	Mean	SD	t value
Global Impairment							
Preschool	628	1.74	.55	602	1.55	.50	5.85****
1st grade	392	1.84	.77	383	1.54	.66	5.63****
2nd grade	426	2.02	.78	412	1.58	.70	8.36****
3rd grade	341	1.97	.76	328	1.69	.73	4.77****
4th grade	158	1.96	.77	159	1.58	.69	4.58****
Referral							
Preschool	621	.20	.17	600	.15	.15	2.69***
1st grade	403	.38	.48	388	.24	.43	4.26****
2nd grade	433	.57	.50	416	.36	.48	6.12****
3rd grade	344	.56	.50	326	.38	.48	4.67****
4th grade	159	.58	.49	165	.36	.48	4.05****

Note.—Preschool scores were averaged over all preschool rating occasions. High scores on Global Impairment indicate poor functioning in the classroom; high scores on Referral indicate that therapeutic or remedial intervention is recommended or actually taking place.

***$p \leqslant .01$.
****$p \leqslant .001$.

former were rated, on average, close to moderately-well functioning while the latter were rated, on average, between moderately-well and well functioning throughout the five-year period of the study. All sex differences were significant at the .001 level.

The grade-to-grade changes are shown in Table 6.5 The boys were significantly more impaired at each grade level in elementary school than during the preschool period, and they were significantly more disturbed in second and third grade than in first grade, with the difference between first and fourth grades approaching significance ($p \leqslant .1$). The differences between second grade and subsequent scores were not significant, indicating that the rising level of pathology peaked at the end of second grade.

In the case of the girls, the only significant change in the ratings occurred in third grade when Global Impairment was

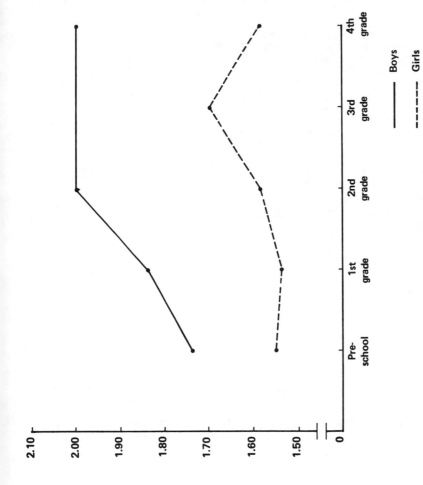

FIG. 5. Global Impairment as a function of age.

Table 6.5 Age Differences on Global Impairment and Referral

Sex and grade level	Mean diff.	t value Preschool versus	Mean diff.	t value 1st grade versus	Mean diff.	t value 2nd grade versus	Mean diff.	t value 3rd grade versus
Part A: Global Impairment								
Boys								
1st grade	.095	−2.45**						
2nd grade	.277	7.16****	.182	4.29****				
3rd grade	.229	5.40****	.134	2.73***	−.048	−1.07		
4th grade	.214	3.47****	.119	1.79	−.063	−0.95	−.078	−1.23
Girls								
1st grade	−.010	−0.29						
2nd grade	−.030	−0.90	.040	1.03				
3rd grade	.131	3.28***	.149	3.33****	.109	2.72***		
4th grade	.029	.53	.039	.67	−.001	−0.02	−.110	−1.97*
Part B: Referral								
Boys								
1st grade	.179	7.31****						
2nd grade	.320	13.07****	.191	6.04****				
3rd grade	.363	12.10****	.184	5.31****	−.007	−0.23		
4th grade	.387	9.39****	.208	4.65****	−.017	−0.40	.021	0.51
Girls								
1st grade	.088	5.09****						
2nd grade	.207	9.24****	.119	4.85****				
3rd grade	.223	8.42****	.135	4.50****	0.16	0.56		
4th grade	.204	5.45****	.116	2.90***	−.003	−0.08	−.019	−0.49

*$p \leqslant .05$.
**$p \leqslant .02$.
***$p \leqslant .01$.
****$p \leqslant .001$.

significantly higher than it had been in preschool and in each of the previous elementary school years. In fourth grade a significant improvement in functioning canceled out the third grade deterioration.

Referral

Data in Table 6.4 show that at each age level a significantly larger proportion of boys than girls required treatment. Referral for boys jumped from an average of .20 during the preschool period to .38 at the end of first grade to .57 by the end of second grade. Since the Referral average was based on

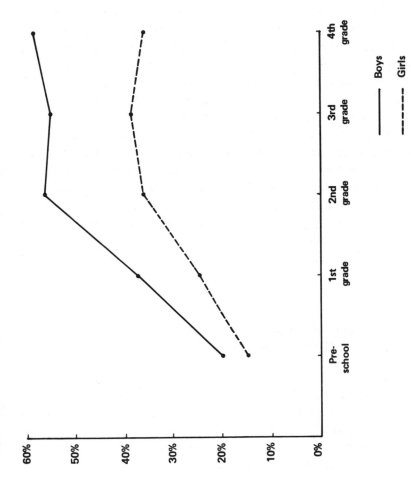

FIG. 6. Referral as a function of age.

dichotomous scores—"no treatment or referral necessary" = 0; "in treatment or referral necessary" = 1—the scores can be translated into percentages. The data mean that the percentage of boys who were perceived to be in need of therapeutic intervention almost tripled in the two years between preschool (20%) and second grade (57%). Thereafter, the percentages remained relatively constant. In other words, from second grade on over half of the boys were referred for treatment by their teachers. The results are displayed in graphic form in Figure 6.

The girls' Referral rate was 15% during the preschool period, 24% at the end of first grade, and 36% at the end of second grade. Thus, the percentage of girls for whom the teachers felt that treatment was indicated more than doubled over the two-year period. After second grade, Referral ratings leveled off.

As may be seen in Table 6.5, the increasing rate of Referral was statistically highly significant. For both sexes all comparisons (a) between the preschool rate and the four subsequent years of elementary school as well as (b) between first grade and the next three years of elementary school were highly significant. No significant differences were found after second grade.

Relationship between syndromes of emotional disturbance and Global Impairment

We wanted to be sure that each of the syndromes was a valid measure of emotional impairment at every age level so that changes in the syndrome scores could be inferred to mean changes in the level of disturbance.

As we suggested in the literature review at the beginning of the chapter, it is possible that scores may increase or decrease because the measuring instrument consists of items that assess behavior traits or problems which are likely to increase or decrease in prevalence during the time period under study. Thus, e.g., if our instruments measured behavior which boys tended to manifest with increasing likelihood as they grew older, the boys' rising level of Apathy-Withdrawal, Anger-Defiance, and Low Task Orientation would be an artifact.

Table 6.6 Correlations between Global Impairment and Syndrome Measures

Sex and grade level	N	Apathy-Withdrawal	Anger-Defiance	Low Task Orientation
Boys				
Preschool	628	.73***	.61***	—
1st grade	392	.52***	.72***	.66***
2nd grade	425	.47***	.74***	.67***
3rd grade	340	.53***	.76***	.67***
4th grade	158	.41***	.65***	.66***
Girls				
Preschool	602	.74***	.56***	—
1st grade	382	.56***	.67***	.54***
2nd grade	411	.57***	.72***	.57***
3rd grade	327	.53***	.62***	.59***
4th grade	158	.68***	.67***	.67***

***$p \leqslant .01$.

One way of subjecting this issue to a test would have been to examine every item on the two elementary school instruments for increase or decrease in prevalence as a function of age.

We decided to approach the question in another way. Since teachers' global ratings have been found to be valid measures of emotional impairment (see chapter 4), we correlated the syndrome scores with the corresponding Global Impairment rating at each age level. We reasoned that the magnitude of the correlations would indicate the degree of validity of the syndrome measure. If a syndrome was composed of items which had low prevalence at a particular age level, it would not be expected to be a valid measure and, therefore, would not correlate highly with Global Impairment. If the correlations were large and remained stable, we could conclude that the syndrome was a valid measure at each age level and that changes in the syndrome scores were in fact indicative of changes in the level of impairment.

The correlations are shown in Table 6.6, separately for boys and girls. Looking at the elementary school data, it may be seen that for boys, the largest correlations were between Anger-

Defiance and Global Impairment (ranging from .65 to .76). Low Task Orientation ranked second in magnitude of correlations ($r = .66$ to $r = .67$) and Apathy-Withdrawal, lowest ($r = .41$ to $r = .53$).

For girls, the largest correlations were also between Anger-Defiance and Global Impairment (ranging from .62 to .72). Apathy-Withdrawal and Low Task Orientation correlations were slightly lower and of approximately equal size (ranging from .53 to .68 for Apathy-Withdrawal and from .54 to .67 for Low Task Orientation).

Thus, for each syndrome, the r values were sizeable and relatively stable and did not vary in a way which would account for changes in the syndrome scores. We concluded that the syndromes were valid measures and that our results reflected actual changes in the level of pathology.

An interesting sidelight emerging from the data in Table 6.6 is the fact that, when preschool and elementary school data are compared, for both sexes, Global Impairment and Apathy-Withdrawal were more strongly correlated in preschool than at any grade level in elementary school while the opposite was true of the relationship between Global Impairment and Anger-Defiance. These results suggest that, in assessing emotional disturbance, the day care teachers were more concerned about passive behavior and less concerned about disruptive behavior than the elementary school teachers.

Summary and comments

The principal findings were:

1. During the preschool period and at each grade level in elementary school boys were rated significantly more disturbed than girls on all three syndrome measures—Apathy-Withdrawal, Anger-Defiance, and Low Task Orientation.

The finding with respect to Anger-Defiance was anticipated and confirmed the results of other researchers cited at the beginning of the chapter. The finding with respect to Apathy-Withdrawal was contrary to expectation and in contrast to research results cited at the beginning of the chapter. However, sex differences on the Apathy-Withdrawal syndrome were considerably smaller than those on Anger-Defiance, actually became nonsignificant in third grade, and were significantly only at the .05 level in fourth grade.

2. As predicted, boys received higher scores than girls on the global ratings—Global Impairment and Referral.

3. In line with our hypotheses on within-sex differences, boys were found to be significantly more impaired on the acting-out syndromes of Anger-Defiance and Low Task Orientation than on the Apathy-Withdrawal syndrome; conversely, girls showed higher levels of Apathy-Withdrawal than of Anger-Defiance and Low Task Orientation. Fourteen of 18 within-sex differences examined during the preschool period and the first four years of elementary school were statistically significant in the expected direction.

Previous investigators (Bower, 1969; Olson, 1930; Rogers, 1942; among others) have speculated that the higher degree of pathology among boys than girls arises from the greater difficulty that boys experience in meeting academic requirements. Our finding that sizeable sex differences exist prior to the onset of formal education makes it unlikely that this is the sole explanation. Since boys scored higher on Anger-Defiance than on Apathy-Withdrawal, the difference may be related to the greater amount of aggression that boys show from early age levels on (see Feshbach, 1970). The greater aggressiveness and boisterousness of boys may be perceived by the day care teachers as an obstacle to the orderly conduct of classroom activities.

4. On each of the three syndromes of disturbance, the boys' scores increased sharply between first and second grade, and they maintained the poor level of functioning both in the third and the fourth grade. On Global Impairment, the boys' scores rose steadily from preschool through second grade and then were relatively constant during the next two years. The percentage of boys for whom Referral was indicated jumped from 20% in preschool to 57% in second grade and remained at this high level thereafter.

The girls showed a marked increase on Apathy-Withdrawal through third grade but no consistent pattern of change on Anger-Defiance, Low Task Orientation, and Global Impairment.

The Referral rate for girls rose from 15% during the preschool period to 36% at the end of second grade; there were no significant changes after second grade.

In sum, for the boys, all measures—syndromes and global ratings—reflected a rising level of disturbance through second grade and continued impairment thereafter; the girls were rated higher only on Apathy-Withdrawal and Referral.

The changes in level of pathology noted in the present study are in sharp contrast to the results of Peterson who, as mentioned earlier, found a decline in Personality problems and Conduct problems from kindergarten to fourth grade.

5. Correlations between each of the syndromes of disturbance and Global Impairment indicated that the syndromes were valid measures and that changes in scores could be interpreted to mean changes in level of impairment.

The magnitude of the correlations between Apathy-Withdrawal and Global Impairment does not support the notion originally put forth by Wickman (1928) and subsequently tenaciously maintained by others (Laycock, 1934; Maes, 1966; McFie, 1934; see also Hunter, 1957, and Schrupp & Gjerde, 1953) that "teachers consider the inhibitive, recessive, unsocial forms of behavior to be of comparatively little consequence while the antisocial, attacking types of conduct are regarded as extremely serious problems" (p. 110). Our data showed, on the contrary, that while the elementary school teachers considered Apathy-Withdrawal less indicative of emotional disturbance than Anger-Defiance, they did take it seriously. The day care teachers in fact characterized inhibited functioning as more impaired than antisocial behavior.

Influence of the social environment. With respect to the two theories mentioned at the beginning of the chapter, the initial spurt in impairment during the school entry phase (propounded by the "crisis theorists") occurred in the present study but the postulated subsequent return to a healthier level of functioning as the children adjust to the school environment was not observed in our data.

Biber and her colleagues' view of the school as a socializing institution precludes predictions unless we know the quality of the school environment. According to this theory, one should not expect an unvarying relationship between age and level of disturbance. Arguing backwards from the theoretical position, the data of the present study suggest that the school environment and the quality of the socio-educational milieu were such that they played a part in the decline in the level of social-emotional functioning.

ACADEMIC ATTAINMENT

Academic attainment variables which were examined for sex and age differences included the Metropolitan Readiness Test, Verbal Achievement, Arithmetic Achievement, Academic Standing, Grade Placement, and Verbal Fluency. As outlined in chapter 4, all measures were obtained during the elementary school period except Verbal Fluency on which data were also collected when the children were in day care.

Sex Differences

Evidence of sex differences in school readiness and school performance has been found in previous studies.

With respect to school readiness, as measured by readiness tests, Pauly (1959) noted that at school entry girls were better prepared than boys to cope with the demands of the academic curriculum. This sex difference was also reported in past editions as well as in the most recent (1976) edition of the Metropolitan Readiness Test. According to Blythe C. Mitchell, Staff Consultant at Harcourt Brace Jovanovich, "the test authors' attitude is that readiness is readiness, and the difference is real. Boys are less ready to learn to read, etc., at entrance to first grade" (Personal communication, May 14, 1975).

On school performance, Anastasi (1958) concluded on the basis of her review of the literature: "In academic work as a whole, girls tend to excel (p. 492). . . . With regard to school progress, girls are consistently more successful than boys. They are less frequently retarded, more frequently accelerated, and promoted in larger numbers than boys. Similarly in school grades, girls excel throughout, even in areas where boys excel on achievement tests" (p. 493).

"Nevertheless, administration of standardized achievement tests reveal sex differences in separate school subjects. On such batteries as the Stanford Achievement Test . . . boys score significantly higher on science, social studies, and arithmetic reasoning; girls in spelling, language usage, and (less consistently) in arithmetic computation" (pp. 492—493).

"In general, girls surpass boys in those school subjects depending largely on verbal abilities . . . . boys excel on those subjects that call into play numerical reasoning and spatial aptitudes" (p. 493).

Tyler (1965) also noted that girls typically outperformed boys in English, spelling, writing, and art while boys outperformed girls in solving problems in arithmetic. Similar conclusions have been drawn in British studies (see Pringle, Butler, & Davie, 1966).

Thus, there appears to be agreement that girls do better than boys on tests and tasks involving verbal skills; in arithmetic sex differences seem to vary with the type of skill tested. We expected our results to be in line with past research findings.

Results

The scores on the academic attainment measures at each age level are displayed in Table 6.7, separately for boys and girls. The significance of the sex differences may be seen in the last column of the table.

Metropolitan Readiness Test

The Metropolitan Readiness Test was administered on one occasion only—namely, when Cohort A entered first grade (the New York City Board of Education discontinued use of the Test). The data in Table 6.7 show that the girls scored significantly higher than the boys. As pointed out above, the sex difference has been noted frequently on this Test although the difference in our sample was somewhat larger than the difference for the standardization sample (see Hildreth, Griffiths, & McGauvran, 1969).

Table 6.7 Academic Attainment as a Function of Sex and Age

Measures	Boys			Girls			Sex diff.
	N	Mean	*SD*	*N*	Mean	*SD*	*t* value
Metropolitan Readiness Test							
1st grade	88	53.16	15.96	95	58.12	13.96	−2.20*
Verbal Achievement							
2nd grade	400	2.60	.98	398	.99		−2.28*
3rd grade	306	3.22	1.26	295	3.55	1.22	−3.26***
4th grade	143	3.90	1.53	152	4.13	1.23	−1.42
Arithmetic Achievement							
3rd grade	269	3.31	1.13	288	3.36	1.06	−0.07
Academic Standing							
1st grade	394	2.09	.77	382	2.41	.69	−6.06****
2nd grade	432	2.06	.75	413	2.22	.72	−3.12***
3rd grade	342	1.96	.78	328	2.21	.74	−4.16****
4th grade	159	1.94	.78	164	2.21	.73	−3.20***
Grade Placement							
2nd grade	477	−0.00	.39	463	0.00	.32	−0.00
3rd grade	359	−0.12	.47	351	−0.04	.37	−2.45**
4th grade	169	−0.19	.53	171	−0.07	.45	−2.19*
Verbal Fluency							
Preschool	628	2.05	.50	602	1.89	.46	5.52****
1st grade	238	1.91	.69	227	1.76	.64	2.39**
2nd grade	434	1.94	.66	416	1.81	.60	3.03***
3rd grade	343	2.03	.63	328	1.89	.61	2.88***
4th grade	158	2.06	.59	165	1.99	.60	0.88

Note. – The Metropolitan Readiness Test was discontinued after Cohort A completed first grade. The Verbal Achievement score is an average of the scores of the Word Knowledge and Reading subtests of the Metropolitan Achievement Tests; the Arithmetic Achievement score is an average of the scores on three Mathematics subtests of MAT. On the other achievement measures, high scores = superior Academic Standing and Grade Placement ahead of age group; low scores = superior Verbal Fluency.

On Verbal Fluency, preschool scores were averaged over all rating occasions. Cohort A was inadvertently omitted from data collection in first grade.

p ≤ .05.
**p* ≤ .02.
***p* ≤ .01.
****p* ≤ .001.

Verbal Achievement

Verbal Achievement was measured by two subtests. Word Knowledge and Reading, of the Metropolitan Achievement Tests. The MAT scores in Table 6.7 are in grade equivalents; the number to the left of the decimal represents the grade level, and the first digit to the right of the decimal represents the number of months since the beginning of the school year. Since these subtests were administered in March of each year during which data were collected, a child in second grade who was performing exactly at grade level would achieve an averaged Word Knowledge and Reading score of 2.7.

As may be seen in Table 6.7, the boys were one month behind grade level in second grade, approximately five months behind in third grade, and eight months behind in fourth grade. Girls were at or slightly ahead of grade level in second grade, one or two months behind grade level in third grade, and six months behind grade level in fourth grade.[17] Sex differences were significant in second and third grade but not in fourth grade.

Arithmetic Achievement

For the Arithmetic Achievement measure, the scores on three subtests (Mathematics Concepts, Mathematics Problem Solving, and Mathematics Computation) of the Metropolitan Achievement Tests were pooled. Since the subtests were administered in February of third grade, a youngster achieving exactly at grade level would obtain an average math score of 3.6. The results indicate that both boys and girls were, on average, approximately two months below grade level in arithmetic skills; there was no significant sex difference.[18]

---

[17]These test scores are not distorted by children who were left behind since each child was kept with the age cohort to which he belonged on the basis of his date of birth.

[18]On the subtests, girls were superior to boys on Mathematics Concepts; boys did better than girls on Mathematics Problem Solving; there was no sex difference on Mathematics Computation. These findings were in line with results cited earlier in the chapter. The pooling procedure had the effect of canceling out the sex differences.

Academic Standing

This was a 3-point scale on which the teacher assessed the child's academic performance relative to that of the rest of the class. A score of 1 meant that the child was in the bottom third of the class, and a score of 3 indicated that the child was in the top third of the class.

Sex differences. As shown in Table 6.7, the boys were rated somewhat above average in first grade; the scores dropped a small amount each year until in fourth grade, the boys were just a little below average.

In first grade, the girls' performance level was about halfway between those of the middle and bright groups in the class; in second grade, the scores declined slightly and then stabilized so that from second through fourth grades the girls' scores stood consistently somewhat above the midpoint of the scale.

Thus, the girls were always rated higher than the boys, and the difference between the sexes was highly significant at each grade level.

Age differences. The grade differences were tested for significance and, as may be seen in Table 6.8, the boys' third and fourth grade ratings were significantly lower than their first grade score; compared to second grade, the third grade score was significantly lower, with the difference between second and fourth grade approaching significance ($p \leqslant .1$). After third grade, the change was not significant.

In the case of the girls, the differences between the first grade rating and scores at each succeeding grade level were significant at the .01 level or better. Thereafter, changes were minimal.

Grade Placement

This score indicated whether a child was in the appropriate grade for his age (coded 0), skipped a grade (plus scores reflecting the number of grades skipped), or repeated a grade (minus scores depending on the number of grades he had been left behind).

It is apparent from Table 6.7 that neither boys nor girls showed any deviation from the appropriate grade placement at the end of second grade when these data were collected for the

Table 6.8 Age Differences on Academic Standing, Grade Placement, and Verbal Fluency

Sex and grade level	Mean diff.	*t* value	Mean diff.	*t* value	Mean diff.	*t* value	Mean diff.	*t* value
	Preschool versus		1st grade versus		2nd grade versus		3rd grade versus	
Part A: Academic Standing								
Boys								
2nd grade			−.033	−0.80				
3rd grade			−.132	−2.81***	−.099	−2.21*		
4th grade			−.154	−2.27*	−.121	−1.87	−.022	0.36
Girls								
2nd grade			−.196	−4.90****				
3rd grade			−.207	−4.41****	−.011	−0.24		
4th grade			−.201	−3.35***	−.005	−0.08	.006	−0.09
Part B: Grade Placement								
Boys								
3rd grade					−.115	−5.13****		
4th grade					−.187	−4.83****	−.072	−2.08*
Girls								
3rd grade					−.040	−2.31*		
4th grade					−.070	−2.02*	−.030	−1.00
Part C: Verbal Fluency								
Boys								
1st grade	−.138	−3.56****						
2nd grade	−.111	−3.34***	.027	0.58				
3rd grade	−.017	−0.51	.121	2.33**	.094	2.51**		
4th grade	.011	0.22	.149	−	.122	2.39**	.028	0.55
Girls								
1st grade	−.135	−3.18***						
2nd grade	−.084	−2.80***	.051	1.14				
3rd grade	−.004	−0.01	.131	2.52**	.080	2.00*		
4th grade	.097	2.02*	.232	−	.181	4.27***	.101	1.91

Note.—On Academic Standing and Grade Placement, minus scores = lower level of achievement; on Verbal Fluency, minus scores = improvement. On Verbal Fluency, a comparison between first and fourth grade scores was not possible because Cohort A was not rated on this measure in first grade.

*$p \leqslant .05$.
**$p \leqslant .02$.
***$p \leqslant .01$.
****$p \leqslant .001$.

first time. In third grade boys were kept back more frequently than girls, and the trend became more pronounced the following year. Sex differences were significant in third and fourth grades.

The decline in the boys' Grade Placement score, representing an increase in the number of boys who were not promoted, was highly significant ($p \leqslant .001$) in both third and fourth grades (see

Table 6.8). For girls, the differences between second grade and each of the next two grades were significant but at a lower level ($p \leqslant .05$), and the difference between third and fourth grade scores was not significant. Thus, the evidence indicates that boys were left behind in increasing numbers as the years went by whereas the number of girls who failed rose more gradually and only until third grade.

Verbal Fluency

The 4-point scale ranged from "superior" = 1 to "minimal or no speech" = 4. It is evident from data in Table 6.7 that the boys were rated slightly below average each year of data collection while the girls were generally rated slightly above average. On four of the five rating occasions, the difference in male-female scores was statistically significant.

Both sexes showed an interesting and roughly similar curvilinear pattern: There was improvement on Verbal Fluency in the first two grades as compared to the preschool period, followed by deterioration in third and fourth grades in comparison to second grade. At the end of the fourth year of elementary school, Verbal Fluency returned to approximately the level prevailing during the preschool period: As may be seen in Table 6.8, the initial increase and subsequent decline in Verbal Fluency scores were significant for both sexes.

Summary and comments

The principal findings were:

1. It is clear that, in terms of academic proficiency and cognitive functioning, going to school is for these children not the useful experience that it ought to be. As measured by the Metropolitan Readiness Test and the verbal subtests of the Metropolitan Achievement Tests, the youngsters were performing close to national norms at the beginning of their school career; however, by fourth grade the girls were six months behind national norms and the boys, eight months.

The decline in the test scores is in line with yearly data published by the New York City Board of Education for all the city's schools and is apparently a trend found in most metropolitan school systems, as has been documented by Coleman (1966) and Sexton (1961), among others.

The children scored approximately two months below grade level when the arithmetic subtests of the Metropolitan Achievement Tests were administered in third grade. They showed deterioration on the Academic Standing measure (through third grade for boys, through second grade for girls). Grade Placement scores revealed a trend, especially pronounced for boys, toward being left behind.

Verbal Fluency was the only measure on which the children showed a gain after entering elementary school, suggesting that the experience initially provided a stimulus to verbal interaction and expression. The fact that the ratings reverted to the level prevailing before the children started first grade further attests to the deleterious effect of the school experience.

2. As anticipated on the basis of past research findings, girls outperformed boys on all but one of the achievement measures. The Metropolitan Readiness Test scores showed that they were better prepared for school than boys. Girls were superior to boys on the verbal subtests of the Metropolitan Achievement Tests (there was no sex difference on the arithmetic subtests). The teachers rated girls higher than boys on Academic Standing and Verbal Fluency, and the incidence of having to repeat a grade was lower among girls than boys.

Representativeness of the sample. By comparing the results we obtained on the Metropolitan Readiness Test with the scores of the population on whom the Test was standardized (the Harcourt Brace Standardization Sample consisted of 12,000 children from diverse walks of life), we can examine the representativeness of our sample.

In the present study the boys obtained an average score of 53 and the girls, an average score of 58. According to Hildreth et al., a total score between 45 and 63 is considered average and acceptable for entry into first grade. These authors present tables, based on the Harcourt Brace Standardization Sample, from which percentile ranks can be computed. In terms of percentile ranks, the boys' score was at the 46th percentile and the girls', at the 57th percentile; the percentile rank of the combined group was 51. Thus, our sample seemed to be just about average.

CONCLUSIONS

It is an accepted maxim that progress in school has practical implications for successful integration into adult society. The damaging effect of school attendance on both the social-emotional functioning and academic attainment of the children in the present study is, therefore, alarming. An appalling picture of increasing emotional impairment and educational backwardness emerges from the results reported in this chapter.

The boys fared worse than the girls: Their social-emotional functioning deteriorated markedly during the first two years of elementary school when they were rated by their teachers as significantly more disturbed on each of five criterion measures. In the next two years there was some leveling off but no improvement.

The boys' scholastic performance declined steadily during each of the first four grades. This is not to imply that they did not gain any language or arithmetic skills but they obviously learned less than they should have, and this is especially debilitating in a culture that places a high premium on education and intellectual achievements.

Among girls, the lowered level of social-emotional functioning was characterized principally by a steady increase in apathetic and withdrawn behavior through third grade and a steep rise in the rate of referrals through second grade. A trend toward underachievement was clearly evident although less severe than for the boys.

There may be more than coincidence in the fact that social-emotional functioning and academic attainment both worsened. The data did not show a 1:1 parallel since in the case of the boys, e.g., learning deficit increased through the fourth year of elementary school whereas the major increase in emotional impairment had taken place by the end of the second grade. However, the stabilization of the impairment measures may have been a function of the frame of reference of the rater, i.e., the teacher.

At each grade level, a teacher uses the behavior of the other children in the class as a yardstick in assessing health or disturbance. Therefore, age differences, even where they exist, are hard to demonstrate. The fact that age differences showed up during the first few years of elementary school indicates that the changes in social-emotional functioning must have been massive. It is likely that further changes would have been noted if the teachers had used a frame of reference broader than their own classroom or if we had had the luxury of independent observers.

The concurrent increase in emotional problems and academic deficiencies cannot be dismissed lightly. It seems plausible to assume that if curricula and teaching styles were more imaginative and appealing, the children's social-emotional (as well as cognitive) functioning would improve. As we have speculated previously (Kohn, 1975; Kohn & Rosman, 1974), there is probably a link between the dimension, Interest-Participation versus Apathy-Withdrawal, and the extent to which the environment is stimulating or boring. In the present study both boys and girls were rated more impaired on this dimension over the course of time.

According to Jerome Colligan, Coordinator of City-Wide Testing (Personal communication, October 20, 1975), the New York City Board of Education, in an informal survey, has identified a number of schools which maintain a high level of academic achievement in spite of the fact that they are slum schools in which one usually finds very poor scholastic performance. It would be interesting to compare the levels of Apathy-Withdrawal, Anger-Defiance, and Low Task Orientation in these schools with levels prevailing in slum schools where children underachieve. We hypothesize that principals and teaching staffs in the former schools provide an effective learning climate and creative instructional materials which foster a high degree of Interest-Participation.

The substantial increase in the percentage of children perceived to require therapeutic intervention is an indication of how overwhelmed the teachers must feel in the face of rising levels of impairment and declining levels of academic performance. Since Referral and Global Impairment are strongly correlated and since Global Impairment is a highly valid measure, the sizeable referral rate should be taken very seriously: The children referred for treatment are in fact disturbed.

The question arises whether these day care children may have been a deviant group, more likely to show impairment and underachieve than their non-day care peers in elementary school. Indications are that they were not a deviant group. First, in elementary school the teachers' frame of reference was not limited to day care children, and both boys and girls were rated, on average, moderately-well functioning or better in first grade. Second, the study sample was average with respect to the Metropolitan Readiness Test scores; and third, girls performed at and boys close to grade level at the first administration of the verbal subtests of the Metropolitan Achievement Tests in second grade. Of course, we do not know whether a comparison group of non-day care children would have exhibited less deterioration in social-emotional functioning and/or scored higher on the academic attainment measures.

CHAPTER 7

Epidemiology and Longitudinal Persistence of Emotional Impairment

We will address ourselves to two issues in this chapter:

1. The relationship between emotional impairment and the sociocultural matrix in which the child is embedded, with specific emphasis on the extent to which emotional impairment in childhood is associated with disadvantaged status;

2. The longitudinal persistence of emotional impairment, with specific emphasis on the extent to which a given syndrome remains stable over time.

Epidemiology of Emotional Impairment

As pointed out in chapter 1, there is considerable evidence that among adults (age 20 and over) prevalence of emotional impairment varies inversely with social status (see Dohrenwend & Dohrenwend, 1969). For example, in the classic study by Faris and Dunham (1939) a high prevalence rate of schizophrenia was found in Chicago's inner city with its heavy concentration of slums and skid rows. Since mental health and social status are concurrent phenomena, however, causal inferences are not easily drawn: Emotional impairment may result in low social status or "disadvantaged status" may lead to emotional disorder.

Let us define our terms: "Status" encompasses the notion of class level, based on socioeconomic considerations such as occupation, education, income, and amount and kind of power. Max Weber has stated (see Gerth & Mills, 1946, pp. 186–187) that there are bases other than social class for determining place in the social structure, e.g., the amount of honor or prestige associated with any quality shared by a plurality. In our society race is one such quality, ethnicity another. Following the ideas propounded by Weber, we intend the term, "status," to cover not only the concept of social class but also of race and ethnicity. Thus, when we speak of "disadvantaged" status in the present investigation, we are referring to individuals who are at a low social class level or belong to a racial or ethnic minority group.

The relationship between low socioeconomic status and marital instability has been repeatedly noted in the literature. Lower-class families are frequently broken by separation, desertion, divorce, or death. Therefore, in the present study disrupted family life was also considered a characteristic of "disadvantaged status."

There are two major theories about the cause-effect relationship between emotional impairment and social status (Dohrenwend & Dohrenwend, 1969). According to the "drift" or "social selection" hypothesis, those who are too disturbed to make their way in society drift into low-paying jobs and low-income neighborhoods; their unfavorable economic circumstances are a consequence of their emotional impairment.

Since evidence for this theory can appear only after the young have left the shelter of home and school and entered the labor market, i.e., have begun to establish their own place in society, the social selection hypothesis is not a plausible one for children. A disturbed child does not drift to disadvantaged parents. Therefore, this theoretical formulation was not applicable in the present study.

According to the "social causation" hypothesis, the circumstances of lower-class existence are so harsh and uncertain, events so unpredictable, family life so disorganized, and family and work roles so marginal that emotional disturbance is produced or accentuated by the difficult and stressful life situation.

Vivid accounts of the ways in which deleterious conditions impinge on the lower-class and minority-group child have been drawn by such authors as Sexton (1961), who particularly emphasized the harmful effects of the child's school life, and Srole et al. (1962) who presented an extensive review of the effects of disadvantaged status on family life, personality development, self-concept, and ego-development. Speaking almost interchangeably of the slum child and the lower-class child, they stated: "The selected pieces of evidence . . . reveal a life setting for the slum-level child heavily weighted with impoverishing burdens and deprivations of body, mind, and spirit, to an extent well beyond the nurturing environment of the middle-class child and far beyond that of the 'cushioned' upper-class child" (p. 198).

"In many areas of his experience the lower-class child encounters the contempt, implicit but palpable, in the nonverbal behavior of others who think of him in the symbolism of such words as rubbish, scum, dregs, riff-raff, and trash. These devastating judgments inevitably force their way into his own self-evaluation processes" (p. 198).

Thus, the social causation hypothesis suggests, almost demands, that the relationship between disadvantaged status and emotional impairment be observable in the early years of life; it would not be at all plausible to assume that the scars resulting from childhood deprivation and insult would be invisible throughout childhood only to appear full-blown in adult life.

On the other hand, to obtain evidence linking children's emotional impairment to their parents' disadvantaged status would be only a first step in proving the social causation hypothesis. The relationship might also be due to genetic or other biological factors. Inclusion of these types of variables would have required a different design and methodology—complications with which we were not prepared to deal in the present investigation. In the present study we were content to determine whether emotional impairment was related to disadvantaged status in the early and middle years of childhood, i.e., between the ages of 3 and 10.

Longitudinal Persistence of Emotional Impairment

As noted in chapter 1, there are conflicting opinions among clinicians about the longitudinal persistence of emotional impairment. One school of thought assumes that disturbance in childhood tends to become chronic, that hope for remission or recovery is slight, and, therefore, these clinicians consider early signs of emotional impairment as premonitory. The other school of thought views disturbance in childhood as a transient phenomenon which frequently disappears as the child grows older, and, therefore, these clinicians do not believe that early impairment is inevitably the precursor of later impairment.

There is a paucity of empirical data; existing research results have not been conclusive. Except for the work of Macfarlane et al. (1954), follow-up studies which yielded evidence of persistence of pathology focused on clinical samples of severely disturbed children (see chapter 2).

We were interested in the question of persistence of emotional impairment in "normal" children. Furthermore, we were not concerned so much with persistence of overall severity of disturbance as with persistence of specific syndromes; e.g., would a child who was rated high on Apathy-Withdrawal at one age score high on the same syndrome a few years later or would the child be just as likely to score high on Anger-Defiance or Low Task Orientation as he grew older? In other words, did each of the three syndromes describe a unique pattern of behavior which remained stable over time?

We tested longitudinal persistence in two ways. First, we selected two prediction periods: (a) a longer period, from preschool through the fourth grade of elementary school—a time span of approximately three and a half years, and (b) a shorter period, from early elementary school to later elementary school—a time span of approximately two years. Our major interest was in the longer period since it represented a more decisive test of the longitudinal persistence hypothesis. We performed the shorter-term within-elementary school analysis primarily to examine the uniqueness of Low Task Orientation, which was not assessed during the preschool period. Because of the high correlation between Anger-Defiance and Low Task Orientation (see Table 4.2), we felt it important to determine whether these were different though strongly related measures of the same syndrome or whether each was a unique syndrome. In addition, we wanted to ascertain to what extent the magnitude of the predictions of persistence would be enhanced when (a) the time span was shorter, (b) there was no change in environment (from day care to elementary school), and (c) there was no change in rating instruments (from Kohn instruments to Peterson and Schaefer instruments).

Second, we studied longitudinal persistence by correlating data from each age level with data from every later age level. The objective was to determine the effect of time on the magnitude of (a) the same-syndrome (e.g., Apathy-Withdrawal to Apathy-Withdrawal) correlations as compared to (b) the cross-syndrome (e.g., Apathy-Withdrawal to Anger-Defiance) correlations. This approach was expected to yield further and more detailed information both on stability of functioning and the feasibility of early identification of children who are at risk of later disturbance.

Major Hypotheses

The major hypotheses were that:

1. The sociocultural matrix in which the child is embedded affects his social-emotional functioning; specifically, emotional impairment is a function of disadvantaged status.

2. Early emotional impairment is predictive of later emotional impairment, and furthermore, the specific type of impairment the child shows at one age level will persist as he grows older.

3. Early emotional impairment is predictive of later emotional impairment over and above the demographic variables, i.e., after

the demographic variables have been removed as a source of variability.

4. When demographic variables and early emotional impairment are taken jointly to predict persistence of disturbance, the magnitude of the relationship will be greater than when the demographic variables are used alone.

More specific hypotheses will be spelled out later in the chapter.

Methods of Data Analysis

The data analytic techniques best suited to test the hypotheses were correlational and hierarchical multiple regression techniques. The correlational technique is one of the simplest ways of determining relationships between variables; a correlation states to what extent a given variable covaries with a second variable. For example, in this analysis we wished to determine to what extent emotional impairment was related to social class.

In the hierarchical multiple regression technique, equal emphasis is placed on "hierarchical" and "multiple." The "multiple" aspect is useful when a given outcome arises from several causes or antecedents, and the researcher wants to determine the extent to which the aggregate effect of the predictor variables can explain the dependent variables. For example, in this analysis we wished to see the joint effect of demographic and preschool social-emotional variables on later emotional impairment.

The "hierarchical" aspect consists of introducing the variables in a sequence (i.e., in a hierarchical way) and permits the researcher to hold some variables constant while he examines the effect of other variables. For example, of the two classes of predictor variables, the demographic data can be introduced into the equation before the preschool social-emotional measures; with demographic variables "partialed out," i.e., controlled for, information is obtained on the extent to which preschool emotional impairment predicts later emotional impairment over and above demographic status.

The same logic applies to the variables within each class of predictor variables. For example, among demographic variables the effect of race or ethnicity is often difficult to interpret because these variables may be confounded with social class. Thus, black subjects may do poorly on a given test not necessarily because of their minority-group status but because they may be lower-class. The effect of race, unconfounded by social class, can be determined with the hierarchical technique by introducing social class before race into the regression equation and thereby removing the variance accounted for by social class.

Each variable or group of variables that is introduced is defined as a set. Stated in other words, statistical control is effected by introducing successive sets of variables into the equation. The proportion of variance of the dependent variables accounted for by each successive set is determined after the variance accounted for by the preceding set(s) has been removed. Each set of variables thus acts as a statistical control for the subsequent set. (For further clarification, it should be pointed out that variables in the preceding sets as well as the remaining variables within the same set are partialed out from one another.) The sequential order of the sets is governed by the specific hypotheses being tested. The cumulative contribution of all sets represents the total amount of variance of the outcome variables accounted for by the predictor variables.

In presenting the results, the terms, "variance," "percentage of variance," and "incremental variance," will be encountered. "Percentage of variance" is a measure of how much information about the dependent variable has been gained from the independent variable. If we cannot account for any variance at all, we have no information; if we can account for 100% of the variance, we have enough information to make perfect predictions. In practice we usually find something in between these two extremes. In a great deal of psychological research we are satisfied if we can account for 2% of the variance; that is usually sufficient to obtain a statistically significant result (see Cohen, 1969).

"Incremental variance" refers to the amount of additional information gained whenever a new variable or set of variables is added to the prediction equation. It represents the extent to which the prediction of the criterion variables has been improved by the addition of this variable or set of variables. The statistical significance of each amount of incremental variance can be calculated to determine whether the finding is a chance result or whether the amount is greater than would be expected by chance.[19]

In order to test the hypotheses and to determine the independent and joint effects of the demographic and social-emotional variables, a very large number of data analyses could have been carried out. For example, with preschool demographic and social-emotional variables as the independent variables, we could have constructed separate hierarchical multiple regression equations using either first, second, third, or fourth grade social-emotional measures as the dependent variables; or, using first grade data as the independent variables, we could have predicted to emotional impairment at each of the later grade levels. In the end, all of these regression equations would have been tiresomely repetitious, and costs would have been prohibitive.

We made the following choices: (a) For the longer period, from preschool through fourth grade, predictions were made from the child's social-emotional functioning in day care (averaged over all rating occasions) to the child's social-emotional functioning in elementary school (averaged over all rating occasions).[20] (b) For the shorter period, from early to later elementary school, predictions were made from early elementary school (grades 1 and 2 averaged) to later elementary school (grades 3 and 4 averaged).

---

[19] The reader interested in a more detailed and technical explanation is referred to Cohen (1968). Cohen has demonstrated the equivalence of multiple and partial regression (MR), on the one hand, and analysis of variance and covariance, on the other.

[20] The decision to pool all elementary school scores derived from uncertainty about the likelihood of longitudinal persistence. As the zero-order correlations later showed, these doubts were not justified. With hindsight, we regret that we did not predict from preschool to fourth grade.

For the comparisons between one age level and every other age level, we did not use the hierarchical multiple regression technique but examined the unaveraged correlations at each grade in elementary school.

The data analysis was divided into several parts; the procedures, specific hypotheses, and results will be presented in the next five sections of this chapter.

PART A: FROM PRESCHOOL THROUGH FOURTH GRADE OF ELEMENTARY SCHOOL

The purpose of this analysis was to study the relationship between the children's behavior patterns in preschool and their functioning during the first four years of elementary school. For this analysis the sample was limited to Cohort A since this was the only age group which was followed for the entire five-year period of the study.

Variables

Dependent variables

The dependent or outcome variables were the elementary school measures of emotional impairment—namely, Apathy-Withdrawal, Anger-Defiance, Low Task Orientation, Global Impairment, and Referral, each averaged across the four grade levels to obtain maximally stable measures for the longitudinal predictions.

Studies establishing the validity of teachers' global assessments were cited in chapter 4. We saw in chapter 5 that Apathy-Withdrawal and Anger-Defiance differentiated normal from disturbed children. In this analysis global measures were used as criterion variables because we felt that the extent to which the preschool syndrome scores predicted to global ratings completed several years later would constitute additional evidence that the syndromes were valid indicators of emotional impairment.

Independent variables

There were two classes of independent or predictor variables: demographic data and the preschool measures of emotional impairment.

The demographic variables included age, sex, and the three indices relevant to disadvantaged status: social class (as measured by mother's education), race-ethnicity, and family intactness.

The preschool measures of emotional impairment were the two syndromes, Apathy-Withdrawal and Anger-Defiance, and the two global measures, Global Impairment and Referral. The global measures were thus used in two ways: as dependent variables, to gain further evidence as to the validity of the syndrome measures; as independent variables, to test the assumption that the syndromes accounted for most of the variance of emotional impairment and that, once the syndromes had been partialed out, the global ratings would no longer be strong predictors of later disturbance. This point will be elaborated on presently.

The predictor variables were introduced in stepwise fashion in successive sets, as outlined in the section on Methods of Data Analysis. The sets, the reasons for their place in the array, and the hypotheses related to them will now be described.

Definition of Sets and Related Hypotheses

Demographic data sets

The demographic variables were introduced prior to the preschool social-emotional measures to avoid false or misleading conclusions. For example, there may be a correlation between healthy social-emotional functioning in preschool and healthy social-emotional functioning in elementary school because a child may come from a "privileged" background which fosters emotional well-being at both points of time in his life. Since demographic variables influence functioning at both age levels, the correlation may be spurious.

There were two sets containing demographic data:

Set 1: Demographic variables. Four variables were included in the first set—age at onset of study, sex, social class, and family intactness. Age trends and sex differences have already been reported in chapter 6. Age and sex were used here primarily as control variables; their effects were removed prior to examining the remaining variables.

(a) Age. Because of the relatively narrow age range of Cohort A at the outset of the study (subjects were between 59 and 70 months old), we expected age to account for relatively little variability of the criterion measures.

(b) Sex. We anticipated sex differences on the global measures and on two of the syndromes, Anger-Defiance and Low Task Orientation, with boys showing considerably more impairment than girls. We looked for only slight, if any, sex differences on Apathy-Withdrawal.

(c) Social class. In past research on adults, emotional impairment has frequently been found to be related inversely to social class. According to Dohrenwend and Dohrenwend (1969), when global or undifferentiated emotional disturbance was used as the criterion, a higher prevalence rate was observed in the lowest social class in approximately 20 out of 25 studies. When specific types of disorders were used as criterion measures, only personality disorders (sociopathy) and possibly schizophrenia were noted more frequently at lower-class than at upper-class levels.

We expected emotional impairment, as assessed both by the global and the syndrome measures, to vary inversely with social class, with lower-class children showing more impairment than lower-middle and middle-class children.

(d) Family intactness. Two kinds of effects on children's social-emotional functioning have been noted in previous studies: 1) a general impairment of functioning and generally higher symptom levels among children from broken than among children from intact homes (Biller, 1970; Langner et al., 1970), and 2) a specific effect, namely, an increase in acting-out and aggressive behavior (Biller, 1970; McCord, McCord, & Thurber, 1962). The break in family life is associated with loss of social control (see Nye, 1958) which in turn is presumed to result in a rise in antisocial behavior.

We expected global as well as specific effects. We predicted that a break in family life would result in higher global impairment, higher incidence of referral, and higher scores on Anger-Defiance and Low Task Orientation. On the other hand, we expected family intactness to have only a minimal effect on Apathy-Withdrawal.

Set 2: Race and ethnic variables. Race and ethnicity were introduced after the other demographic variables to avoid confounding minority-group status with social class and family intactness. We had three ethnic groups in the sample: whites, blacks, and Puerto Ricans. We divided the three groups into two contrasting variables—namely, (a) white versus black and Puerto Rican children, and (b) black versus Puerto Rican youngsters. The first comparison would be informative on the effect of minority-group status; the second would be informative on differences between the two minority groups.

The deleterious effect of minority-group status has been amply documented in a series of studies carried out in the 30's and 40's describing the caste and class systems in the southern United States. For example, in their analysis of social stratification in a major city in the Deep South before World War II, Davis, Gardner, and Gardner (1958) wrote as follows of the distinction between the white and Negro castes: "The 'caste line' defines a social gulf across which Negroes may not pass either through marriage or those other intimacies which Old City calls 'social equality.' A ritual reminder is omnipresent in all relationships that there are two separate castes—a superordinate white group and a subordinate Negro group" (p. 371).

While some of the most formidable barriers between the races are no longer quite as oppressive, qualitatively not that much has changed. Throughout the country blacks and Puerto Ricans, as well as other minority groups such as Indians and Mexican-Americans, still live in the anguish and despair that accompanied the caste system of the old Deep South.

This point of view was reflected in the "war on poverty" during the 1960's. The Joint Commission on Mental Health of Children (1969) stated: "Very early in the Commission's study, it was recognized that the mental health problems of minority-group children are severe enough to warrant special consideration" (p. 215) . . . "Presently, many minority-group children are denied the opportunities to achieve this ideal state of mental health. Only rarely does the child of an ethnic minority escape the damaging effects of racism. Often racism and poverty combine to cripple the minority-group child in body, mind and spirit" (p. 216).

Yet, contrary to the Commission's assertions, epidemiological studies comprising both black and white adults have revealed no clear trend for one or the other group to show a higher rate of disturbance (see Dohrenwend & Dohrenwend, 1969, p. 31).

We hypothesized that black and Puerto Rican children would be significantly more impaired in social-emotional functioning than white children. However, after controlling for social class and family intactness, we expected the magnitude of the correlations to be substantially reduced. We had no hypothesis for the second variable, i.e., the comparison between black and Puerto Rican children.

Preschool emotional impairment sets

There were two sets of emtional impairment variables:

Set 3: Syndrome variables. Apathy-Withdrawal and Anger-Defiance constituted the variables in this set. We expected syndrome persistence over time, i.e., the child who scored high on Apathy-Withdrawal during the preschool period would be rated high on Apathy-Withdrawal during the elementary school period, and the same for Anger-Defiance. Cross-syndrome correlations over time (preschool Apathy-Withdrawal to elementary school Anger-Defiance and vice versa) were expected to be trivially small, if not insignificant.

Schaefer's Factor III, High versus Low Task Orientation, was only assessed after the children had entered elementary school; since Low Task Orientation was strongly correlated with Anger-Defiance, we predicted that the child who was rated disturbed on Anger-Defiance in preschool would be rated disturbed on Low Task Orientation during the middle years of childhood.

It was expected that both preschool syndromes would be strongly related to the two global measures. We assumed that if a child scored high on either Apathy-Withdrawal or Anger-Defiance or both in preschool, he was likely to exhibit signs of disturbance and be a candidate for referral as he grew older.

Set 4: Global variables. The last set contained Global Impairment and Referral, two variables which we expected to be very broadgauged, covering just about anything that teachers might consider as indicative of disturbed functioning. We assumed that Apathy-Withdrawal and Anger-Defiance accounted for a large proportion of emotional impairment in children; if this assumption was correct, the global ratings would add relatively little variance over and above that accounted for by the two preschool syndromes. If, however, Apathy-Withdrawal and Anger-Defiance represented limited facets of emotional impairment, the global ratings would contribute a large amount of additional information to the prediction equation.

We hypothesized that the fourth set containing the two preschool global ratings would account for little incremental variance of the later emotional impairment measures and that the magnitude of the correlations would be sharply reduced after the syndromes had been partialed out.

Results

The results are presented in Table 7.1 and 7.2. Table 7.1 shows the relationship between the demographic and preschool social-emotional variables and the elementary school gobal measures; Table 7.2 shows the relationship between the same predictor variables and the elementary school syndrome measures. The data appear under column headings, $\Delta R^2\%$, r_o, and r_p. $\Delta R^2\%$ represents the incremental amount of information which a set of variables contributed to the prediction equation. Zero-order correlations (r_o) indicate the magnitude of the direct relationship between an independent and a dependent variable when the effect of other variables has not been held constant. Partial correlations (r_p) show the magnitude of the relationship between the independent and dependent variable after variables in the same and previous sets have been statistically controlled for.

The final lines in each table show the total amount of variance which all the independent variables taken together account for in the criterion variable (total $R^2\%$) as well as the multiple correlation coefficients when all the variables are used as predictors simultaneously (R). Since the multiple regression approach always tends to inflate the amount of variance accounted for, the corrected R^2% and the corrected R, adjusted to offset this bias (McNemar, 1969), are also presented.

In this section of the chapter (Part A) and in the next (Part B), our focus will be on (a) how much variance each set accounted for, (b) what the significant zero-order correlations between individual variables were, and (c) what variables remained significant after partialing. The data on total variance will be discussed in a later section (Part D) of the chapter.

Relationship between predictor variables and global measures

We now turn to an examination of Table 7.1.

Set 1: Demographic variables. The variables in set 1 collectively accounted for a significant amount of variance of Global Impairment (12.0%) and Referral (8.7%).[21] However, only one variable within the set—sex—showed significant correlations (zero-order and partial) with both global measures. The direction of the relationship indicates that, as predicted, boys were rated as significantly more poorly functioning than girls and were referred for treatment significantly more often than girls.

Contrary to our expectations, the data provided no evidence that children from lower-class or broken families functioned more poorly or were more in need of referral than children from families at higher social class levels or from families that were intact.

Set 2: Race and ethnic variables. This set did not account for any significant amount of variance of either criterion measure; neither zero-order nor partial correlations were significant. There was no evidence whatsoever that children from minority backgrounds were emotionally more disturbed or in greater need of intervention than white children. The hypothesis was not confirmed.

---

[21] As expected, age accounted for little variability of the dependent variables and will not be discussed further in this section (Part A) or the next (Part B).

Table 7.1 Relationship between Demographic and Preschool Social-Emotional Variables and Elementary School Global Measures

Demographic & Preschool social-emotional variables	df	Elementary school global measures (Grades 1–4 averaged)					
		Global Impairment			Referral		
		ΔR²%	r_o	r_p	ΔR²%	r_o	r_p
Set 1	4/290	12.0***			8.7***		
Age			−.08	−.13		.01	−.03
Sex			−.32***	−.33***		−.29***	−.29***
Social class			−.04	−.04		−.06	−.04
Family intactness			.03	.05		−.02	.04
Set 2	2/288	0.8			0.4		
White versus Others			−.04	−.03		.00	.01
Black versus Puerto Rican			.04	.08		.02	.07
Set 3	2/286	15.1***			16.6***		
Preschool Apathy-Withdrawal			.36***	.23***		.36***	.24***
Preschool Anger-Defiance			.40***	.27***		.41***	.27***
Set 4	2/284	2.8**			10.1***		
Preschool Global Impairment			.47***	.19**		.51***	.19**
Preschool Referral			.28***	.03		.57***	.27***
Total R²%	10/284	30.7***			35.8***		
R		.55			.60		
Corrected R²%		28.3			33.5		
Corrected R		.53			.57		

Note.—ΔR²% = (ΔR² × 100) which shows the increment in variance contributed by each set; r_o = zero-order correlation; r_p = partial correlation.

Demographic variables were scored as follows: sex: 1 = male, 2 = female; social class: mother's education on a 7-point scale based on Hollingshead's system from 1 = under seven years' schooling to 7 = some graduate education; family intactness: 1 = both parents at home, 2 = broken home; white versus others: 1 = white, −1 = black or Puerto Rican; black versus Puerto Rican: 1 = black, 0 = white, −1 = Puerto Rican.

For all measures of social-emotional functioning, high scores = disturbance.

*p ≤ .05.
**p ≤ .01.

Set 3: Syndrome variables. The two variables in this set accounted for a significant amount of variance of the two dependent variables, 15.1% of Global Impairment and 16.6% of Referral. These percentages are impressive and indicate clearly that the relationship between early and later social-emotional functioning is not due to a spurious correlation resulting from common demographic variables. In other words, there is no merit to the argument that a child from a privileged background may be rated well functioning in preschool and also several years later because, at both rating occasions, the socioeconomic circumstances of his life were conducive to emotional health.

The partial correlations between preschool Apathy-Withdrawal and the two elementary school global ratings (r_p = .23 with Global Impairment and r_p = .24 with Referral, $p \leqslant .001$) were very similar in magnitude to the partial correlations between preschool Anger-Defiance and the two elementary school global measures (both r_p = .27, $p \leqslant .001$). These results suggest that (a) as anticipated, a child who scored high on either syndrome in day care was likely to be perceived emotionally impaired and in need of treatment in elementary school, and (b) the chances of being rated emotionally impaired and needing referral were about the same regardless of which syndrome the child exhibited during the preschool period.

Set 4: Global variables. The amount of variance added by the last set was statistically significant: The amount accounted for by Global Impairment was small (2.8%) but the amount accounted for by Referral was more substantial (10.1%).

The four zero-order correlations among the variables were all highly significant. In particular, the results indicate that disturbance in day care was predictive of disturbance several years later (r_o = .47, $p \leqslant .001$) and that need of treatment during the preschool period was likely to persist in elementary school (r_o = .57, $p \leqslant .001$).

After partialing, the correlations became considerably smaller: Preschool Global Impairment was still significantly, but much more modestly, correlated with elementary school Global Impairment and Referral (both r_p = .19, $p \leqslant .01$). Preschool Referral was still significantly related to elementary school Referral (r_p = .27, $p \leqslant .001$) but no longer showed a significant correlation with Global Impairment (r_p = .03, *n.s.*).

Thus, in line with our assumption, the amount of variance for which the preschool global variables accounted and the magnitude of the correlations were sharply reduced after the syndrome measures had been partialed out.

Relationship between predictor variables and syndrome measures

Examination of Table 7.2 shows the following results:

Set 1: Demographic variables. The variables in set 1 collectively accounted for a significant amount of variance of each of the three syndromes, 4.1% of Apathy-Withdrawal, 12.1% of Anger-Defiance, and 11.0% of Low Task Orientation.

The only significant r_p values were between sex and the syndrome measures; correlations of $r_p = -.34$ ($p \leqslant .001$) with Anger-Defiance and $r_p = -.31$ ($p \leqslant .001$) with Low Task Orientation indicated that boys were rated higher than girls on these syndromes. A smaller ($r_p = -.14$) but still significant ($p \leqslant .05$) relationship between sex and Apathy-Withdrawal showed boys to be somewhat more impaired on that dimension than girls.

The hypothesis that emotional impairment would vary inversely with social class was not confirmed. A small but significant zero-order correlation ($r_o = -.12$, $p \leqslant .05$) between social class and Apathy-Withdrawal was in line with expectations; however, after statistically controlling for the other variables in set 1, it was no longer significant. Low social class status did not predict either to Anger-Defiance or to Low Task Orientation. Thus, as with the global ratings, the data failed to show any significant relationship between emotional impairment in the middle years of childhood and parents' social class level.

Also contrary to expectation, family intactness was not significantly correlated with Anger-Defiance or Low Task Orientation.

Set 2: Race and ethnic variables. Set 2 accounted for a small but significant portion of variance of Anger-Defiance (2.0%). There was also a significant zero-order correlation with Anger-Defiance, suggesting that white children were rated lower on the syndrome than black and Puerto Rican children; but the correlation was small ($r_o = -.11$, $p \leqslant .05$) and, after partialing,

Table 7.2 Relationship between Demographic and Preschool Social-Emotional Variables and Elementary School Syndrome Measures

Demographic & Preschool social-emotional variables	df	Elementary school syndrome measures (Grades 1–4 averaged)								
		Apathy-Withdrawal			Anger-Defiance			Low Task Orientation		
		$\Delta R^2\%$	r_o	r_p	$\Delta R^2\%$	r_o	r_p	$\Delta R^2\%$	r_o	r_p
Set 1	4/290	4.1*			12.1***			11.0***		
Age			-.07	.08		.00	-.05		-.07	-.12*
Sex			-.13*	-.14*		-.34***	-.34***		-.30***	-.31***
Social class			-.12*	-.11		.00	-.01		-.01	-.02
Family intactness			.07	-.05		.06	.08		.07	.09
Set 2	2/288	0.0			2.0*			0.4		
White versus Others			.00	.00		-.11*	-.10		-.03	-.03
Black versus Puerto Rican			-.04	.02		.08	.08		.02	.04
Set 3	2/286	18.3***			19.0***			14.5***		
Preschool Apathy-Withdrawal			.44***	.44***		.21***	.00		.22***	.05
Preschool Anger-Defiance			.04	-.15**		.51***	.44***		.43***	.36***
Set 4	2/284	2.2*			2.2*			1.4*		
Preschool Global Impairment			.37***	.15**		.44***	.18**		.38***	.14**
Preschool Referral			.21***	.03		.22***	-.04		.20***	-.02
Total $R^2\%$	10/284	24.7***			35.2***			27.3***		
R		.49			.59			.52		
Corrected $R^2\%$		22.4			33.3			25.1		
Corrected R		.47			.58			.50		

Note.—$\Delta R2\% = (\Delta R^2 \times 100)$ which shows the increment in variance contributed by each set; r_o = zero-order correlation; r_p = partial correlation.

Demographic variables were scored as follows: sex: 1 = male, 2 = female; social class: mother's education on a 7-point scale based on Hollingshead's system from 1 = under seven years' schooling to 7 = some graduate education; family intactness: 1 = both parents at home, 2 = broken home; white versus others: 1 = white, −1 = black or Puerto Rican; black versus Puerto Rican: 1 = black, 0 = white, −1 = Puerto Rican.

For all measures of social-emotional functioning, high scores = disturbance.

*$p \leqslant .05$.
**$p \leqslant .01$.
***$p \leqslant .001$.

149

no longer significant. Thus, the evidence supported only weakly the hypothesis that during the middle years of childhood minority-group children would be more impaired in their social-emotional functioning than white youngsters.

Set 3: Syndrome variables. The set containing the preschool measures of emotional impairment accounted for a significant amount of variance of all three elementary school syndromes. Percentages ranged from 14.5% to 19.0% and thus were higher than the proportion of variance contributed by the demographic variables.

At the zero-order level, the correlations showed a relatively high degree of specificity: Preschool Apathy-Withdrawal, but not preschool Anger-Defiance, was significantly correlated with elementary school Apathy-Withdrawal. Although both preschool syndromes were significantly related to elementary school Anger-Defiance, the Anger-Defiance versus Anger-Defiance correlation ($r_o = .51$, $p \leqslant .001$) was appreciably higher than the Apathy-Withdrawal versus Anger-Defiance correlation ($r_o = .21$, $p \leqslant .001$). The preschool measures showed approximately the same pattern of r_o values to elementary school Low Task Orientation as to elementary school Anger-Defiance.

After partialing, the evidence of persistence of type of impairment became even clearer. With one exception, all correlations showed the 1:1 relationship that was predicted from preschool to the middle years of childhood: The child who was rated high on Apathy-Withdrawal in day care scored high on this syndrome during the first four years of elementary school, and the child who was assessed impaired on Anger-Defiance during the preschool period was rated high on that syndrome and on Low Task Orientation in elementary school. The exception was a small but significant inverse correlation between preschool Anger-Defiance and elementary school Apathy-Withdrawal, indicating that the child who was rated cooperative and compliant (the healthy pole of the Anger-Defiance dimension) in day care showed a significant tendency to be shy and withdrawn during the elementary school period.

Set 4: Global variables. This set accounted for a small but significant amount of additional variance (1.4% to 2.2%) of each of the three elementary school syndrome measures.

At the zero-order level, correlations between preschool Global Impairment and the three syndromes were moderate in size (ranging from .37 to .44, $p \leqslant .001$); the partial correlations were considerably lower (ranging from .14 to .18, $p \leqslant .01$). The direction of the correlations indicates that the child who was seen by his day care teacher as poorly functioning scored higher on each syndrome pattern (i.e., less healthy) in elementary school than the child who had been perceived as well functioning during the preschool period.

The r_o values between preschool Referral and the three syndromes ranged from .20 to .22 and were significant at the .001 level. These findings suggest that the child who was thought to be in need of therapy in preschool scored higher on all three syndrome measures in later years than the child who did not appear to require treatment. After all other independent variables had been partialed out, the correlations became very small and were no longer significant.

Thus, at this point in the prediction equation, Global Impairment and Referral contributed only small or insignificant increments to the variance of the syndrome measures.

Summary

Demographic variables. The principal findings were:

1. The two sets containing demographic data jointly accounted for 9.1%–12.8% of the variance of the global ratings and 4.1%–14.1% of the variance of the syndrome measures.

2. Sex was the most potent of the demographic predictor variables. As expected, boys received significantly higher scores than girls on the global ratings and were significantly more impaired than girls on Anger-Defiance and on Low Task Orientation. Unexpectedly, boys also scored significantly higher than girls on Apathy-Withdrawal but sex differences on that syndrome were smaller than those on the acting-out behavior patterns.

3. None of the hypotheses as to the effect of disadvantaged status on emotional impairment were fully confirmed. With two exceptions, there was no evidence that social class, family intactness, or race-ethnicity were predictive of disturbance

during the middle years of childhood. The exceptions were significant zero-order correlations between (a) low social class and Apathy-Withdrawal, and (b) minority-group status and Anger-Defiance. However, the correlations were no longer significant after partialing.

Emotional impairment variables. The principal findings were:

1. In line with expectations, preschool emotional impairment was predictive of later emotional impairment; not only did the preschool measures have predictive power after the demographic variables had been statistically controlled for but they accounted for a larger proportion of the variance of the criterion measures than the demographic data. The figures were 17.9%–26.7% for the variance of the global ratings and 15.9%–20.5% for the variance of the syndrome measures.

2. There was a strong relationship between the preschool syndrome measures and the later global ratings, as hypothesized; the chances of being rated emotionally impaired and in need of referral in elementary school were about the same whether the child exhibited apathetic-withdrawn or angry-defiant behavior in preschool.

3. As expected, impairment on specific syndromes persisted. Cross-syndrome correlations were consistently lower than syndrome-to-syndrome correlations and after partialing only one was significant—namely, an inverse relationship between preschool Anger-Defiance and elementary school Apathy-Withdrawal which suggested that children who were cooperative and compliant in preschool were apathetic and withdrawn during the elementary school period.

4. As anticipated, the preschool global variables accounted for only modest amounts of incremental variance after the syndrome measures had been partialed out. Zero-order correlations among the global ratings and between global ratings and syndromes were sizeable and significant but r_p values were considerably lower. The data supported our view that the syndrome measures encompassed most of the behavior traits that teachers considered symptomatic of emotional impairment.

PART B: FROM EARLY ELEMENTARY SCHOOL TO LATER ELEMENTARY SCHOOL

The purpose of this analysis was to compare the children's behavior patterns at the beginning of their school career with their social-emotional functioning a few years later. Data for Cohorts A and B were available for this analysis.

Variables

The dependent variables were the elementary school measures of emotional impairment—Apathy-Withdrawal, Anger-Defiance, Low Task Orientation, Global Impairment, and Referral. For each of these measures, the third and fourth grade scores were averaged.[22]

The independent variables consisted of the demographic data and the elementary school measures of emotional impairment, each of the latter averaged over first and second grade.

Definition of Sets and Related Hypotheses

Relationship between predictor variables and global measures

Five sets were introduced into the hierarchical multiple regression equation, as follows:

Sets 1 and 2. These sets, containing the demographic variables, and the related hypotheses were identical to those used in the analysis described in Part A.

Set 3. This set was composed of two syndrome measures, Apathy-Withdrawal and Anger-Defiance. We again expected a strong relationship to the global ratings.

Set 4. This set consisted of the third syndrome measure, Low Task Orientation, not assessed during the preschool period. The purpose of placing Low Task Orientation in a separate set was to determine whether it accounted for any variance of the global measures after Apathy-Withdrawal and Anger-Defiance had been partialed out.

[22] For Cohort B, only third grade measures were available.

Set 5. Global Impairment and Referral again made up the last set, and we again anticipated that, at this point in the equation, they would contribute little incremental variance to the prediction of the later measures and that the correlations would diminish considerably after the effect of the syndrome variables had been controlled for.

Relationship between predictor variables and syndrome measures

Four sets were used in this analysis:

Sets 1 and 2. As before, these sets consisted of the demographic variables.

Set 3. All three elementary school syndrome measures were placed in this set; the purpose of putting all the syndromes into the same set was to test the hypothesis that, at the point when the three syndromes were partialed out from one another, each early syndrome would predict uniquely to the corresponding later syndrome.

Set 4. This set contained the global variables.

Results

Relationship between predictor variables and global measures

Data showing the relationship between the independent variables and the elementary school global measures are shown in Table 7.3.

Set 1: Demographic variables. Set 1 variables again accounted for a significant amount of variance of both dependent variables (4.7% of Global Impairment and 5.1% of Referral). As in the preschool through fourth grade analysis, the highest correlations were with sex, and the direction of the correlations indicates that boys were more severely impaired and were more likely to be referred for treatment than girls.

There was a small but significant partial correlation between social class and Global Impairment, lending some support to the

Table 7.3 Relationship between Demographic and Early Elementary School Social-Emotional Variables and Later Elementary School Global Measures

Demographic & Early elementary school social-emotional variables	df	Later elementary school global measures (Grades 3 and 4 averaged)					
		Global Impairment			Referral		
		$\Delta R^2\%$	r_o	r_p	$\Delta R^2\%$	r_o	r_p
Set 1	4/599	4.7***			5.1***		
Age			.08*	.08*		.11**	.11**
Sex			−.16***	−.15***		−.18***	−.18***
Social class			−.07	−.08*		−.05	−.05
Family intactness			.11**	.12**		−.06	.07
Set 2	2/597	0.7			0.5		
White versus Others			−.03	−.01		−.02	.00
Black versus Puerto Rican			.04	.08		.03	.07
Set 3	2/595	18.9***			16.1***		
Apathy-Withdrawal (1g & 2g)			.27***	.16***		.28***	.18***
Anger-Defiance (1g & 2g)			.45***	.37***		.40***	.32***
Set 4	1/594	2.3***			1.6**		
Low Task Orientation (1g & 2g)			.45***	.18***		.39***	.14**
Set 5	2/592	5.0***			5.3***		
Global Impairment (1g & 2g)			.53***	.23***		.51***	.25***
Referral (1g & 2g)			.38***	.06		.32***	.00
Total $R^2\%$	11/592	31.6***			28.6***		
R		.56			.53		
Corrected $R^2\%$		30.3			27.3		
Corrected R		.55			.52		

Note.−$\Delta R^2\%$ = (ΔR^2 × 100) which shows the increment in variance contributed by each set; r_o = zero-order correlation; r_p = partial correlation.

Demographic variables were scored as follows: sex: 1 = male, 2 = female; social class: mother's education on a 7-point scale based on Hollingshead's system from 1 = under seven years' schooling to 7 = some graduate education; family intactness: 1 = both parents at home, 2 = broken home; white versus others: 1 = white, −1 = black or Puerto Rican; black versus Puerto Rican: 1 = black, 0 = white, −1 = Puerto Rican.

For all measures of social-emotional functioning, high scores = disturbance.

1g & 2g = scores from the two grade levels were averaged.

*p ≤ .05.
**p ≤ .01.
***p ≤ .001.

hypothesis that the lower the social class, the poorer the child's emotional functioning.

There was also a small but significant correlation between family intactness and Global Impairment, bearing out the hypothesis that children from broken homes would be more disturbed than children from intact homes.

Neither social class nor family intactness was significantly related to Referral.

Set 2: Race and ethnic variables. This set did not account for any significant amount of variance of either dependent variable nor were any of the correlations significant. The data did not confirm the hypothesis that children from minority backgrounds would be more disturbed than white children.

Set 3: Syndrome variables. Apathy-Withdrawal and Anger-Defiance together accounted for a significant and relatively large amount of variance of Global Impairment (18.9%) and Referral (16.1%), or more than three times as much variance as the demographic variables accounted for. The prediction of a strong relationship between the syndrome measures and the global ratings was confirmed. All correlations were significant; however, the zero-order Anger-Defiance correlations (r_o = .45 for Global Impairment and r_o = .40 for Referral, $p \leqslant .001$) were appreciably higher than the zero-order Apathy-Withdrawal correlations (r_o = .27 for Global Impairment and r_o = .28 for Referral, $p \leqslant .001$). As may be seen in Table 7.3, the r_p values similarly reflected the fact that, although all correlations remained significant, Anger-Defiance was the more important of the two dimensions in determining the teacher's assessment of impairment and need of therapy.

Set 4: High versus Low Task Orientation. This set accounted for a significant but small proportion of the variance of the criterion measures (2.3% of Global Impairment and 1.6% of Referral). In other words, after Apathy-Withdrawal and Anger-Defiance had been controlled for, Low Task Orientation contributed only slightly to the prediction of the global ratings.

The r_o values between the syndrome measure and Global Impairment and Referral were .45 and .39 ($p \leqslant .001$), respectively; the partial correlations were sharply lower, .18 ($p \leqslant .001$) and .14 ($p \leqslant .01$), respectively.[23] The data show that ratings of Low Task Orientation toward the beginning of

---

[23] This large reduction in the magnitude of the partial correlations as compared to the zero-order correlations is undoubtedly due to the fact that the Low Task Orientation variable was preceded by the Anger-Defiance variable in set 3. When all three syndromes, as measured in early elementary school, were introduced simultaneously in set 3, each accounted for about the same amount of variance of Global Impairment (r_p = .16 for Apathy-Withdrawal, r_p = .14 for Anger-Defiance, and r_p = .18 for Low Task Orientation). Compared to data in Table 7.3, Apathy-Withdrawal and Low Task Orientation were unchanged but Anger-Defiance was lower because of the common variance shared with Low Task Orientation. In other words, when examined simultaneously, all three factors contributed equally to the teacher's assessment of impairment.

elementary school predicted to disturbed functioning and need of therapeutic intervention several years later.

Set 5: Global variables. The two early elementary school global measures jointly accounted for a significant though modest amount of variance of later Global Impairment (5.0%) and later Referral (5.3%).

There were significant r_o and r_p values between early Global Impairment and the later global measures, suggesting that the early rating was predictive of disturbed functioning as the child grew older.

Significant zero-order correlations between Referral and the later global variables indicated that the child who required treatment at the beginning of elementary school was likely to be perceived as impaired and requiring treatment at a later age. After partialing, Referral was no longer significantly correlated with the later global variables.

In sum, the findings were in line with expectations.

Relationship between predictor variables and syndrome measures

The findings appear in Table 7.4.

Set 1: Demographic variables. The demographic variables in set 1 collectively accounted for a significant amount of variance of all three syndromes, 1.9% of Apathy-Withdrawal, 6.7% of Anger-Defiance, and 6.8% of Low Task Orientation.

As predicted, boys were significantly more impaired than girls on Anger-Defiance and Low Task Orientation. Sex differences on Apathy-Withdrawal were now so small that they were no longer significant.

The relationship between social class and Apathy-Withdrawal, suggested by the small zero-order correlation found in the preschool through fourth grade analysis, showed up more strongly in the present analysis, with children from lower-class families rated significantly more inhibited in their functioning than children from families higher on the social scale. However, the evidence did not support the hypothesis that lower social class status would also be related to Anger-Defiance and Low Task Orientation.

Table 7.4 Relationship between Demographic and Early Elementary School Social-Emotional Variables and Later Elementary School Syndrome Measures

Demographic & Early elementary school social-emotional variables	df	Later elementary school syndrome measures (Grades 3 and 4 averaged)								
		Apathy-Withdrawal			Anger-Defiance			Low Task Orientation		
		$\Delta R^2\%$	r_o	r_p	$\Delta R^2\%$	r_o	r_p	$\Delta R^2\%$	r_o	r_p
Set 1	4/605	1.9**			6.7***			6.8***		
Age			-.00	-.00		-.02	-.02		-.04	-.05
Sex			-.06	-.06		-.24***	-.24***		-.24***	-.24***
Social class			-.11*	-.12*		-.01	-.03		-.05	-.06
Family intactness			.01	.03		.10*	.10*		.09*	.09*
Set 2	2/603	0.1			1.6**			0.8		
White versus Others			-.02	-.02		-.08	-.05		-.06	-.04
Black versus Puerto Rican			-.02	-.01		.09*	.10*		.01	.07
Set 3	3/600	22.7***			30.5***			28.3***		
Apathy-Withdrawal (1g & 2g)			.47***	.46***		.12**	-.09*		.12**	-.07
Anger-Defiance (1g & 2g)			.13**	-.12**		.60***	.36***		.51***	.12**
Low Task Orientation (1g & 2g)			.18***	.12**		.52***	.10*		.57***	.33***
Set 4	2/598	1.6**			2.0***			1.1**		
Global Impairment (1g & 2g)			.33***	.14***		.53***	.18***		.48***	.13**
Referral (1g & 2g)			.23***	.01		.54***	-.03		.33***	-.01
Total $R^2\%$	11/598	26.2***			50.7***			37.0***		
R		.51			.64			.61		
Corrected $R^2\%$		24.7			39.5			35.7		
Corrected R		.50			.63			.60		

Note. $-\Delta R^2\% = (\Delta R^2 \times 100)$ which shows the increment in variance contributed by each set; r_o = zero-order correlation: r_p = partial correlation.

Demographic variables were scored as follows: sex: 1 = male, 2 = female; social class: mother's education on a 7-point scale based on Hollingshead's system from 1 = under seven years' schooling to 7 = some graduate education; family intactness: 1 = both parents at home, 2 = broken home; white versus others: 1 = white, −1 = black or Puerto Rican; black versus Puerto Rican: 1 = black, 0 = white, −1 = Puerto Rican.

For all measures of social-emotional functioning, high scores = disturbance.

1g & 2g = scores from the two grade levels were averaged.

*p < .05.
**p < .01.
***p < .001.

158

The prediction that children from broken homes would score higher on Anger-Defiance and Low Task Orientation than children from intact homes but that disrupted family life would not be associated with Apathy-Withdrawal was confirmed.

Set 2: Race and ethnic variables. This set accounted for a small but significant portion (1.6%) of Anger-Defiance. While the data showed no differences between white and minority-group children, significant zero-order and partial correlations indicated that black children exhibited angry-defiant behavior to a greater degree than Puerto Rican children.

Set 3: Syndrome variables. The three early elementary school syndrome measures collectively accounted for a significant proportion of variance of each of the later elementary school syndrome measures. With percentage ranging from 22.7% (Apathy-Withdrawal) to 30.5% (Anger-Defiance), the social-emotional variables contributed a considerably larger amount of variance to the prediction equation than the demographic variables.

The data indicated syndrome persistence; cross-syndrome correlations showed a varied pattern. (a) The relationship between early and later Apathy-Withdrawal was specific: r_o = .47 and r_p = 46, both $p \leqslant .001$. At the zero-order level, early Apathy-Withdrawal was significantly related to later Anger-Defiance and Low Task Orientation but correlations were small (both r_o = .12, $p \leqslant .01$). After partialing, the correlation with Low Task Orientation became nonsignificant; the correlation with Anger-Defiance remained significant but underwent a change in direction, indicating that Interest-Participation (the polar opposite of Apathy-Withdrawal) in early elementary school predicted to angry-defiant behavior a few years later.

At the zero-order level, early Anger-Defiance and early Low Task Orientation were significantly related to later Apathy-Withdrawal (r_o = .13, $p \leqslant .01$ for Anger-Defiance and r_o = .18, $p \leqslant .001$ for Low Task Orientation). After partialing, both correlations remained significant: Early Low Task Orientation continued to be linked directly to later Apathy-Withdrawal but a reversal of signs in the Anger-Defiance r_p's suggest that the child who was initially perceived as cooperative-compliant (the healthy pole of the Anger-Defiance dimension) showed recessive behavior as he grew older. The latter finding corresponds to the result obtained in the preschool through fourth grade analysis.

(b) The relationships between early and later Anger-Defiance and early and later Low Task Orientation were not specific, as was to be expected in view of the high correlation between the syndromes.[24] Same-syndrome correlations were r_o = .60 for Anger-Defiance and r_o = .57 for Low Task Orientation, each r_o value significant at the .001 level. But the cross-syndrome correlations were nearly as large, r_o = .51, $p \leqslant .001$ between early Anger-Defiance and later Low Task Orientation and r_o = .52, $p \leqslant .001$ between early Low Task Orientation and later Anger-Defiance. After partialing, however, it became clear that early elementary school Anger-Defiance predicted uniquely to later elementary school Anger-Defiance (r_p = .36, $p \leqslant .001$) and that early Low Task Orientation predicted uniquely to later Low Task Orientation (r_p = .33, $p \leqslant .001$). The cross-syndrome correlations, though still significant, had shrunk considerably (r_p = .12, $p \leqslant .01$ between early Anger-Defiance and later Low Task Orientation and r_p = .10, $p \leqslant .05$ between early Low Task Orientation and later Anger-Defiance).

Thus, the partialing procedure enabled us to establish that even though Anger-Defiance and Low Task Orientation were strongly correlated, the two syndromes measured different facets of disturbed functioning, generated differential predictions regarding longitudinal persistence of emotional impairment, and that, over time, children remained relatively stable on each unique and specific syndrome measure.

Set 4: Global variables. The last set accounted for a small but significant amount of additional variance (1.1% to 2.0%) of each of the three syndrome measures. The zero-order correlations between the global ratings and the syndromes were all respectable-to-moderate in size and significant at the .001 level, indicating that children with high Global Impairment and Referral ratings early in elementary school were likely to show disturbance on all syndromes in later elementary school.

---

[24] Correlations between the two syndromes were r = .78 and r = .73 during the early and later elementary school period, respectively.

After partialing, Global Impairment was still significantly related to each syndrome although the correlations had diminished in size. The r_p values between Referral and the syndromes were now so small that they were no longer significant.

The data confirmed the hypothesis that, with all other variables partialed out, the global measures would add only a small amount of variance to the prediction equation and the magnitude of the correlations would drop sharply.

Summary

Demographic variables. The principal findings were:

1. The two sets containing demographic data jointly accounted for 5.4%–5.6% of the variance of the global ratings and 2.0%–8.3% of the variance of the syndrome measures.

2. Sex was the most potent of the demographic predictor variables. Boys received significantly higher scores than girls on the global measures and were significantly more impaired than girls on Anger-Defiance and Low Task Orientation; however, there was no significant sex difference on Apathy-Withdrawal.

3. The hypotheses relating social class to emotional impairment were partially confirmed: Children from lower-class families were rated significantly more disturbed on Global Impairment and on Apathy-Withdrawal than children from families higher on the social scale. However, the evidence did not support the assumption that lower-class status would also be related to Anger-Defiance and Low Task Orientation.

4. As expected, children from broken families scored significantly higher on Global Impairment, Anger-Defiance, and Low Task Orientation than children from families that were intact; there was no significant difference on Apathy-Withdrawal.

5. The data did not bear out the hypothesis that children from minority-group backgrounds would be more disturbed than white children. However, the results showed that black children scored higher on Anger-Defiance than Puerto Rican children.

Emotional impairment variables. The principal findings were:

1. The early elementary school social-emotional measures accounted for a considerably larger proportion of variance of the

criterion measures than the demographic data: 23.0%–26.2% of the global ratings and 24.3%–32.5% of the syndromes.

2. As anticipated, high scores on each of the three syndromes were predictive of high global ratings; the findings suggest that in elementary school the teachers viewed angry-defiant behavior as more indicative of disturbed functioning and need of referral than apathetic-withdrawn behavior.

3. Impairment on Apathy-Withdrawal persisted but there were interesting deviations from expectations with respect to the cross-syndrome correlations. (a) An inverse correlation between early Apathy-Withdrawal and later Anger-Defiance indicated that a small but significant number of children who were rated as showing interest and involvement in activities and peers in early elementary school were rated as exhibiting angry-defiant behavior a few years later. (b) An inverse correlation between early Anger-Defiance and later Apathy-Withdrawal suggested that a small but significant number of youngsters whom the teachers perceived as cooperative and compliant toward the beginning of elementary school showed inhibited functioning in subsequent years. (c) While early Apathy-Withdrawal was not significantly related to later Low Task Orientation, early Low Task Orientation was significantly associated with later Apathy-Withdrawal.

4. Impairment on the Anger-Defiance syndrome persisted.

5. Low Task Orientation was found to be a unique pattern of behavior, strongly related to but distinctive from Anger-Defiance. Early Low Task Orientation predicted to later Low Task Orientation.

6. In line with expectations, the global measures accounted for only small amounts of incremental variance, and correlations with the criterion measures declined markedly after the syndromes had been statistically controlled for. The evidence confirmed the assumption that the syndromes were highly inclusive measures of what teachers regarded as disturbed behavior in children.

PART C: FURTHER EXAMINATION OF THE RELATION-SHIP BETWEEN DEMOGRAPHIC VARIABLES AND EMOTIONAL IMPAIRMENT MEASURES

The specific hypotheses relating the variables relevant to disadvantaged   status   (social   class,   family   intactness,   and race-ethnicity) to emotional impairment were only mildly supported in the two data analyses reported so far. Therefore, we undertook another analysis to determine whether more clear-cut findings would emerge when the data were examined separately by sex and at successive age levels.

For this purpose we drew on the two missing-data correlation matrices (one containing the boys' data; the other, the girls' data) which we had generated prior to carrying out the multiple hierarchical regression analysis (for procedural details, see section on Sample Attrition in chapter 4). From these matrices we extracted the correlations between the demographic variables and the emotional impairment measures. In order to smooth out the data, all preschool emotional impairment measures had been averaged for the preschool period, and all elementary school impairment variables had been averaged through second grade for all subjects, through third grade for Cohorts A and B, and through fourth grade for Cohort A.

Results

The data are presented in Table 7.5. For the sake of clarity, only the correlations which were significant at the 5% level or better are shown. The differences between the boys' and girls' correlations were tested for significance of differences by means of the t test, and the level of significance of the differences may be seen in Table 7.6.

In looking at Table 7.5, two major results stand out:

1. There were a large number of small but significant correlations between social class and emotional impairment for *girls*.

2. There were a large number of small but significant correlations between family intactness and emotional impairment for *boys*.

Social class

For girls, the bulk of the significant correlations were between social class and Apathy-Withdrawal (preschool and elementary school), Global Impairment, and Referral; there was one

Table 7.5 Relationship between Demographic Variables and Social-Emotional Measures: By Sex

Social-emotional measures	N	Boys					Girls				
		Age	Social class	Family intactness	White versus Others	Black versus Puerto Rican	Age	Social class	Family intactness	White versus Others	Black versus Puerto Rican
Preschool											
Apathy-Withdrawal	597	—	—	—	—	—	—	-.12**	—	—	—
Anger-Defiance	592	—	—	.11*	—	—	—	—	.12**	—	—
Elementary school											
Apathy-Withdrawal											
to 2nd grade	482	—	—	—	—	—	—	-.11*	—	—	—
to 3rd grade	379	—	—	—	—	—	—	-.14*	—	—	—
to 4th grade	189	—	—	—	—	—	—	-.18**	—	—	—
Anger-Defiance											
to 2nd grade	482	—	—	.14**	—	—	—	.11	—	-.17***	.12**
to 3rd grade	379	—	—	.17***	—	—	—	—	—	-.14*	.17***
to 4th grade	189	—	—	.20**	—	—	—	—	—	—	.15*
Low Task Orientation											
to 2nd grade	482	—	—	.12**	—	—	—	-.11*	—	-.12*	.12*
to 3rd grade	379	—	—	.15**	—	—	—	—	—	—	—
to 4th grade	189	—	—	.22**	—	—	—	—	—	—	—
Global Impairment											
to 2nd grade	473	—	—	.14**	—	—	—	-.11*	—	—	—
to 3rd grade	377	—	—	.13*	—	—	-.12*	-.11*	—	—	—
to 4th grade	188	-.15*	—	.20**	—	—	—	-.16**	—	—	—
Referral											
to 2nd grade	473	—	—	—	—	—	-.12*	-.11*	—	—	—
to 3rd grade	377	—	—	—	—	—	-.14*	-.24***	—	—	—
to 4th grade	188	—	—	.15*	—	—	—	—	—	—	—

Note. — Demographic variables were scored as follows: social class: high score = high social class; family intactness: 1 = both parents at home, 2 = broken home; white versus others: 1 = white, -1 = white versus others; white versus Puerto Rican: 1 = black or Puerto Rican; black versus Puerto Rican: 1 = black, 0 = white, -1 = Puerto Rican. For all measures of social-emotional functioning, high scores = disturbance.

To 2nd grade, to 3rd grade, to 4th grade = scores from that grade and from the preceding grades were averaged. Average scores to 2nd grade include all three Cohorts; to 3rd grade, Cohorts A and B; to 4th grade, Cohort A only.

*$p \leq .05$.
**$p \leq .01$.
***$p \leq .001$.

significant correlation each between social class and Anger-Defiance and social class and Low Task Orientation.

The magnitude of the correlations increased slightly with age: for Apathy-Withdrawal, from $r = -.12$ and $r = -.11$ in preschool and second grade, respectively, to $r = -.18$ in fourth grade; for Global Impairment, from a nonsignificant correlation in second grade to $r = -.16$ in fourth grade; for Referral, from a nonsignificant correlation in second grade to $r = -.24$ in fourth grade.

For boys, none of the correlations between social class and impairment was significant.

When the boys' and girls' correlations were tested for significance of differences, seven were found to be statistically significant at the 5% level or better. As may be seen Table 7.6, the significant differences occurred mostly in the third and fourth grades.

Family intactness

For boys, family intactness was significantly related to Anger-Defiance (preschool and elementary school), Low Task Orientation, Global Impairment, and, to a lesser extent, Referral. The impact of broken family life tended to increase with age: Correlations with Anger-Defiance rose from $r = .11$ and $r = .14$ in preschool and second grade, respectively, to $r = .20$ in fourth grade; with Low Task Orientation, from $r = .12$ in second grade to $r = .22$ in fourth grade; with Global Impairment, from $r = .14$ in second grade to $r = .20$ in fourth grade; and with Referral, from nonsignificant to $r = .15$ by the end of fourth grade.

For girls, the only significant correlation between family intactness and emotional impairment occurred at the preschool level. Like the boys, girls from broken homes scored higher than girls from intact homes on Anger-Defiance. During the elementary school period none of the correlations was significant.

When the boys' and girls' correlations were tested for significance of differences, four were found to be significant at the 5% level or better; all occurred between second and fourth grade.

Table 7.6 Relationship between Demographic Variables and Social-Emotional Measures: Significance of Differences between Boys' and Girls' Correlations

Social-emotional measures	Age	Social class	Family intactness	White versus Others	Black versus Puerto Rican
Preschool					
Apathy-Withdrawal	--	−	−	−	−
Anger-Defiance	−	−	−	−	−
Elementary school					
Apathy-Withdrawal					
to 2nd grade	−	−	−	−	−
to 3rd grade	−	$p \leqslant .01$	−	−	−
to 4th grade	−	$p \leqslant .05$	−	−	−
Anger-Defiance					
to 2nd grade	−	−	−	−	$p \leqslant .05$
to 3rd grade	−	−	$p \leqslant .05$	$p \leqslant .05$	−
to 4th grade	−	−	−	−	−
Low Task Orientation					
to 2nd grade	−	−	−	−	−
to 3rd grade	−	$p \leqslant .02$	−	−	−
to 4th grade	−	−	$p \leqslant .05$	−	−
Global Impairment					
to 2nd grade	−	−	$p \leqslant .01$	−	−
to 3rd grade	$p \leqslant .001$	$p \leqslant .001$	−	−	−
to 4th grade	$p \leqslant .05$	$p \leqslant .001$	−	−	−
Referral					
to 2nd grade	−	−	−	−	$p \leqslant .001$
to 3rd grade	−	$p \leqslant .02$	−	−	−
to 4th grade	−	$p \leqslant .001$	$p \leqslant .02$	$p \leqslant .05$	$p \leqslant .05$

Note.—To 2nd grade, to 3rd grade, to 4th grade = scores from that grade and from the preceding grades were averaged. Average scores to 2nd grade include all three Cohorts; to 3rd grade, Cohorts A and B; to 4th grade, Cohort A only.

Race-ethnicity

The data point to some interesting but less conclusive results on the relationship between minority-group status and emotional impairment. Girls from minority groups scored higher than white girls on Anger-Defiance in third and in fourth grade and on Low Task Orientation in third grade; black girls showed a similar pattern vis-a-vis Puerto Rican girls. In other words, as measured by the amount of acting-out behavior, black girls were more disturbed than either white or Puerto Rican girls.

We found no significant racial or ethnic differences among the boys.

Tests of significance of differences between the boys' and girls' correlations produced five differences significant at the 5% level or better; three of these were in the Referral ratings (even though zero-order correlations had been nonsignificant).[25]

Summary

When the data were examined separately by sex and at cumulative successive age levels, a clearer picture emerged regarding the relationship between disadvantaged status and emotional impairment than had been found in the previous regression analyses. The principal findings were:

1. Girls accounted for the association between low social class level, as measured by mother's education, and Apathy-Withdrawal and Global Impairment observed in the early to later elementary school prediction period. The results also revealed an inverse relationship between social class and Referral, indicating that teachers perceived lower-class girls to be more in need of therapeutic intervention than girls at higher class levels. The sex differences were significant.

2. Boys were largely responsible for the relationship (noted in the within-elementary school analysis) between disrupted family life and Anger-Defiance, Low Task Orientation, and Global Impairment. The differences between the sexes were significant.

In the present study more than half of the families were broken due to father absence. The differential effect of social class on girls and family intactness on boys may be explained by the absence of or deficiency in the same-sex role model: Girls are more disturbed when the mother is educationally handicapped; boys are more impaired when there is no consistently present male figure with whom to identify.

[25] The meaning of the significant differences is as follows: White boys were less likely to be referred than minority-group boys; white girls were more likely to be referred than minority-group girls. Black boys were more likely to be referred than Puerto Rican boys; black girls were less likely to be referred than Puerto Rican girls. These results suggest that among boys, blacks were seen in need of referral the most and whites, the least; among girls, whites were seen in need of referral the most and blacks, the least.

3. The correlations between social class and disturbance for girls and between family intactness and pathology for boys gave some indication of age trends: The disadvantaged status variable seemed to have an increasingly damaging effect as the child grew older.

4. Girls accounted for the finding made in the within-elementary school analysis that black children showed greater impairment than Puerto Rican children on Anger-Defiance. A new result, in the expected direction, was that girls from minority groups were more disturbed on Anger-Defiance and, to some extent, on Low Task Orientation than white girls. In general, the racial and ethnic variables appeared to have the weakest predictive value of the three disadvantaged status variables.

PART D: PREDICTIVE POWERS OF DEMOGRAPHIC AND EMOTIONAL IMPAIRMENT VARIABLES

In presenting our findings, we have so far focused on the relationship between a specific predictor variable and a specific criterion measure. In this section we will discuss the effect of the demographic variables as a group and the emotional impairment measures as a group and analyze the separate and joint value of the two classes of variables in predicting later emotional impairment.

Results

Table 7.7 contains data drawn from Tables 7.1 through 7.4. Data in Part A of Table 7.7 indicate the total variance for which the class of demographic and the class of emotional impairment variables accounted, separately and jointly, during the period, from preschool through fourth grade, and data in Part B of the table represent comparable data for the period, from early to later elementary school. It should be noted that the percentages shown for the emotional impairment measures are the variance that this class of variables contributed after the demographic variables had been partialed out.

Table 7.7 Percentage of Variance Accounted for by Demographic and Social-Emotional Variables, Separately and Jointly, in the Prediction of Later Emotional Impairment

Variables	df	Global Impairment	Referral	Apathy-Withdrawal	Anger-Defiance	Low Task Orientation
Part A: Preschool through fourth grade prediction period[a]						
Total demographic	6/288	12.8%	9.1%	4.1%	14.1%	11.4%
Total preschool social-emotional[b]	4/284	17.9%	26.7%	20.5%	21.2%	15.9%
Total all variables	10/284	30.7%	35.8%	24.7%	35.2%	27.3%
Total all variables, corrected for shrinkage		28.3%	35.5%	22.4%	33.3%	25.1%
Part B: Early to later elementary school prediction period[c]						
Total demographic	6/597	5.4%	5.6%	2.0%	8.3%	7.6%
Total early elementary social-emotional[b]	5/592	26.2%	23.0%	24.3%	32.5%	29.4%
Total all variables	11/592	31.6%	28.6%	26.2%	40.7%	37.0%
Total all variables, corrected for shrinkage		30.3%	27.3%	24.7%	39.5%	35.7%

[a]Relevant measures from the four rating occasions in elementary school were averaged.

[b]The variance shown for social-emotional variables is after demographic variables have been partialed out.

[c]Relevant measures from third and fourth grade were averaged.

Separate effect of each class of variables

The demographic variables accounted for small-to-modest proportions of variance, ranging from 4.1% to 14.1% in the longer prediction period and from 2.0% to 8.3% in the shorter prediction period. These percentages lose some of their luster when it is recalled that a large share of the variability was contributed by one variable—sex.

The emotional impairment measures accounted for 15.9% to 26.7% of the variance from preschool through fourth grade and for 23.0% to 32.5% from early to later elementary school. Thus, they contributed considerably larger amounts than the demographic data to the prediction of later emotional impairment. Had the demographic variables not been partialed out to avoid spurious results, the social-emotional measures would have accounted for an even more substantial share of the variance.

Joint effect of classes of variables

The demographic and social-emotional variables together accounted for a large proportion of the variance of the outcome variables: between 24.7% and 35.7% for the preschool through fourth grade period and between 26.7% and 40.7% for the within-elementary school period. The gain in predictive power resulting from combining the two classes of variables was not as substantial as had been anticipated, however, since sex was the only demographic variable that consistently showed a strong effect.

The amount of variance accounted for in the five criterion measures—Global Impairment, Referral, Apathy-Withdrawal, Anger-Defiance, and Low Task Orientation—is not large enough to make predictions for individual children; however, percentages are sufficiently high to pinpoint groups of children likely to be disturbed at a later age.

PART E: EXAMINATION OF SAME-SYNDROME AND CROSS-SYNDROME LONGITUDINAL CORRELATIONS

This analysis had a two-fold purpose: (a) to compare the magnitude of the same-syndrome longitudinal correlations with the magnitude of the cross-syndrome longitudinal correlations; and (b) to give the reader the more conventional type of data with which he may be more familiar from other studies. Sample size varied with the time span under study; the range was from $N = 1,232$ in preschool to $N = 246$ from second to fourth grade.

Results

In contrast to data presented in previous sections of this chapter, the figures in Table 7.8 are unaveraged zero-order correlations. For the same-syndrome comparisons we will discuss (a) data along the horizontal rows to obtain an indication of longitudinal persistence as time span between rating occasions increased, and (b) data along the first diagonal to determine stability of functioning when time lapse between measurements

Table 7.8 Longitudinal Correlations of Apathy-Withdrawal, Anger-Defiance, and Low Task Orientation

	Apathy-Withdrawal					Anger-Defiance					Low Task Orientation			
	Pre-school	Grade				Pre-school	Grade				Grade			
		1st	2nd	3rd	4th		1st	2nd	3rd	4th	1st	2nd	3rd	4th
Apathy-Withdrawal														
Preschool		.37	.36	.33	.28	.35	.13	.11	.12	.17	.13	.14	.15	.17
1st grade			.48	.39	.37		.32	.11	.05	.12	.26	.14	.08	.10
2nd grade				.47	.43			.36	.14	.11		.28	.12	.12
3rd grade					.50				.37	.15			.30	.12
4th grade										.38				.36
Anger-Defiance														
Preschool						.47	.44	.35	.36		.37	.37	.35	.31
1st grade							.58	.47	.48		.70	.47	.42	.40
2nd grade								.59	.51			.75	.50	.42
3rd grade									.60				.78	.60
4th grade														.75
Low Task Orientation														
1st grade												.54	.44	.47
2nd grade													.49	.42
3rd grade														.57
4th grade														

Note.—$N = 1,232$ within preschool, $N = 780$ within 1st grade, $N = 856$ within 2nd grade, $N = 670$ within 3rd grade, $N = 323$ within 4th grade.

$N = 780$ from preschool to 1st grade, $N = 856$ from preschool to 2nd grade, $N = 670$ from preschool to 3rd grade, $N = 323$ from preschool to 4th grade.

$N = 664$ from 1st grade to 2nd grade, $N = 484$ from 1st grade to 3rd grade, $N = 265$ from 1st grade to 4th grade.

$N = 564$ from 2nd grade to 3rd grade, $N = 246$ from 2nd grade to 4th grade.

$N = 289$ from 3rd grade to 4th grade.

was held constant at one year.[26] To study cross-syndrome patterns, we will compare the correlations between different syndromes when ratings were obtained at the same point in time with correlations between different syndrome measures taken at increasing intervals of time.

Stability of same-syndrome longitudinal correlations

Apathy-Withdrawal. It may be seen in the top horizontal row of the column headed, "Apathy-Withdrawal," that the correlation between preschool and first grade Apathy-Withdrawal was $r = .37$; although the correlations between the preschool score and ratings at later grade levels gradually declined, even after a lapse of four years, the fourth grade correlation was still respectable (r

[26] The preschool data were averaged across rating occasions and, therefore, the preschool to first grade data may involve, on average, a longer time lapse than the grade-to-grade data in elementary school.

= .28). All within-elementary school longitudinal correlations also decreased slightly over time.

Data along the first diagonal indicate that, with time span between ratings held constant at one year, the longitudinal correlations within the elementary school period were somewhat larger than the preschool to first grade correlation: first to second grade was r = .48, second to third grade, r = .47, and third to fourth grade, r = .50.

Anger-Defiance. The second set of data in the column headed, "Anger-Defiance," show that the preschool to first grade correlation was r = .47; as the time lapse between ratings rose, the r values became smaller but by fourth grade the correlation with the preschool score was still moderate in size (r = .36). Over time all longitudinal correlations diminished slightly.

Inspection of data along the first diagonal reveals that the one-year within-elementary school correlations were somewhat larger than the preschool to first grade correlation; the range of the within-elementary school correlations was narrow, from r = .58 (first to second grade) to r = .60 (third to fourth grade).

Low Task Orientation. As noted before, scores were not obtained during the preschool period. The third set of data in the column labeled, "Low Task Orientation," indicate the expected pattern—namely, a slight decrease in the size of the correlations as time lapse between rating occasions increased (first to second grade, r = .54; first to fourth grade, r = .47). There were minor fluctuations in the magnitude of the correlations when the time interval between measurements was held constant at one year.

Comparison of syndromes. The data suggest Anger-Defiance to be the most stable of the three syndromes over time: The correlations were somewhat larger than those for Apathy-Withdrawal and slightly larger than those for Low Task Orientation. The latter ranked second in stability: The longitudinal correlations were smaller than the r values of Anger-Defiance but larger than the Apathy-Withdrawal correlations.

Stability of cross-syndrome longitudinal correlations

Apathy-Withdrawal versus Anger-Defiance. The first set of data in the column headed, "Anger-Defiance," show that during the preschool period the correlation between Apathy-Withdrawal and Anger-Defiance was r = .35; however, as the time period between measurements increased, the correlations shrank considerably: r values between preschool Apathy-Withdrawal and first to fourth grade Anger-Defiance scores varied between .11 and .17.

The pattern of sharply declining correlations with the passage of time was evident in each year of elementary school. In first grade the within-grade correlation between the syndromes was r = .32 but the correlations between first grade Apathy-Withdrawal and subsequent Anger-Defiance scores ranged from r = .05 to r .12. Similar results were observed at second and third grade levels.

Apathy-Withdrawal versus Low Task Orientation. The first set of data in the "Low Task Orientation" column reveal that when measures were obtained at the same point in time, the cross-syndrome correlations ranged from r = .26 in first grade to r = .36 in fourth grade. As the time spans between ratings became longer, the cross-syndrome correlations dropped (r = .08 to r = .17).

Anger-Defiance versus Low Task Orientation. The second set of data in the "Low Task Orientation" column indicate that the within-grade r values were substantial (.70 to .78). The between-grade correlations were smaller but remained moderate in size; e.g., the correlation between preschool Anger-Defiance and fourth grade Low Task Orientation was r = .31, between first grade Anger-Defiance and fourth grade Low Task Orientation, r = .40.

Summary

When persistence of type of impairment was assessed in terms of the magnitude of the unaveraged same-syndrome and cross-syndrome longitudinal correlations, the principal findings were:

1. The same-syndrome correlations declined gradually over time but even after a lapse of four years, correlations were still of respectable size, r = .28 for Apathy-Withdrawal and r = .36 for Anger-Defiance. Stability varied somewhat with the

syndrome tested; angry-defiant behavior was found to show the strongest longitudinal persistence.

With time lapse held constant at one year, the within-elementary school correlations were larger than the preschool to first grade correlations.

2. There was a sharp reduction in the size of the cross-syndrome correlations as the time span between ratings increased. Apathy-Withdrawal was moderately correlated with the other two syndromes when measures were obtained at the same point in time but the correlations became small after a lapse of only one year. On the other hand, Anger-Defiance and Low Task Orientation were highly correlated when measures were obtained at the same grade level; although correlations decreased over time, they were still of moderate magnitude three years later.

CONCLUSIONS

Epidemiology of Emotional Impairment

In line with the social causation theory, we had expected to find a relationship between emotional impairment and parent's disadvantaged status. However, the demographic variables accounted for only small-to-modest proportions of the variability of the youngsters' social-emotional functioning in both prediction periods. Moreover, most of the variance was contributed by sex and not by the variables relevant to disadvantaged status. Among the latter, the number of statistically significant partial correlations was small, and they showed up only in the data analysis for the shorter period, from early to later elementary school.

Of the three indicators of disadvantaged status, disrupted family life was the most potent predictor of disturbed behavior in the classroom. In line with expectations, children from broken homes showed anger, frustration, restlessness, and impairment viewed globally to a significantly greater degree than children from intact homes. When the data were analyzed separately by sex and at successive age levels, it turned out that the findings were mainly attributable to the boys' behavior and that pathology became gradually more pronounced as the children grew older.

In the present sample more than 50% of the households were headed by women, and we assume that the boys' disturbed functioning was a consequence of father absence. The finding corresponds to the conclusion reached by Biller (1970) who noted in his review of the literature that girls showed relatively less impairment as a result of father absence than boys.

Social class was not as strong a correlate of emotional impairment as anticipated. As hypothesized, there were significant inverse relationships between social class level and inhibited functioning as well as disturbance seen from a global point of view; but low social class was only very mildly associated with aggressive types of behavior. Data analysis by sex and age showed that the findings applied only to girls and that the link between low social class and submissive behavior became gradually stronger over time.

The study of Shepherd et al. (1971) is of interest here because their results parallel ours, i.e., they found a small but significant correlation between social class and "deviant" behavior in school among girls but not among boys. Other investigators have failed to find a relationship between social class and disturbance in early childhood (see Bennett, 1960; Bower, 1969; Cullen & Boundy, 1966a; Davidson, 1961; Lapouse & Monk, 1964; Mitchell, 1965; Mulligan, 1964; Rutter et al., 1970; von Harnack, 1953).

In a few studies contrary results have been obtained (see Langner, Goff, Greene, Herson, & Jameson, 1970; Langner, Goff, Greene, Herson, Jameson, & McCarthy, 1969; Lurie, 1970; Pringle, Butler, & Davie, 1966; Rogers, 1942). The study by Rogers is open to criticism since the criteria of emotional impairment included measures of educational achievement, and this raises a question because cognitive and emotional functioning do not show the same relationship to social class. Langner and his associates and Lurie dealt with broad age categories and were not concerned with the age level at which the relationship between emotional impairment and social status first becomes apparent. The only serious challenge to our findings is posed by the work of Pringle et al., and the reason for the difference in results is not clear.

In general, the racial and ethnic variables appeared to have even less impact on children's social-emotional functioning than family intactness and social class. Race-ethnicity was examined after the effects of the other demographic variables had been partialed out to avoid spurious results. Based on the significant partial correlations, there was only one finding: Black children were rated significantly more disturbed on Anger-Defiance than Puerto Rican children. When data were broken down by sex and age levels, we discovered that girls accounted for the result. This analysis also showed that both black and Puerto Rican girls were more impaired on Anger-Defiance and, to some extent, on Low Task Orientation than white girls. In other words, the postulated link between minority-group status and mental health variables based on strongly worded views set forth in recent publications (e.g., Joint Commission on Mental Health of Children, 1969; among others), was only mildly supported by the data of the present study.

As noted, the adverse impact of broken family life on the behavior of the boys and of low social class status on the functioning of the girls tended to increase with age. This finding may provide the key to reconciling the virtual absence of a relationship between disadvantaged status and disturbance in early childhood with evident presence of the relationship in adulthood. After the early years of life, the child moves out of the family setting into the street, and "street life" becomes one of the major environmental influences on his development. He enters school where he is exposed to different cultural norms and values and may be treated with suspicion and derision by his teachers and classmates. It is likely that these and other factors in the larger social milieu cumulatively contribute to the emergence of psychopathology.

In the present study the relationship between disadvantaged status and emotional impairment was relatively weak at the preschool level. By fourth grade, when the children were 10 years old, the correlations were stronger though still not very robust. Judging by the slow acceleration in the size of the correlations, it is plausible that the relationships between social status and mental health variables may not reach their full magnitude until adolescence or early adulthood. Research designed to shed light on this hypothesis is urgently needed.

On the basis of our data, we draw the following conclusion about the epidemiology of emotional impairment: Much of what has been generalized about the deleterious effects of disadvantaged status on social-emotional functioning is at best a gross oversimplification of the facts. Sex, age, and syndrome of disturbance have to be specified when linking disadvantaged status and emotional impairment.

The fact that the data provided only sparse support for the social causation hypothesis is not to imply that parents do not exert a strong influence on their children's mental health. Study results attesting to the vital impact of the family setting on the major dimensions of children's social-emotional functioning were reported in chapter 2 (see Hewitt & Jenkins, 1946; Kohn & Rosman, 1971; Morris, Escoll, & Wexler, 1956). The evidence suggests that although the parent-child relationship has a potent effect on social-emotional functioning, it is not class-patterned in a way that makes for a 1:1 relationship between social class and emotional impairment. It may be a stereotyped belief of the middle-class intellectual that lower-class mothers are less loving and less concerned about their children than middle-class mothers.

Longitudinal Persistence of Emotional Impairment

By a variety of tests, the study yielded evidence of persistence of disturbance both from preschool through fourth grade and from early to later elementary school. The social-emotional variables accounted for 16% to 27% of the variance of emotional impairment in the longer prediction period and for 23% to 33% in the shorter period, considerably more than the variance contributed by the demographic variables. These amounts are adequate for the early identification of groups of children who are likely to experience social-emotional difficulties as they grow older.

The results confirmed many of the hypotheses but afforded some surprises. The early syndrome measures predicted to the later global ratings, providing further evidence that each pattern of disturbance was a valid clinical entity. All syndromes remained moderately stable over time, with r_p values ranging from .33 to .46.

Anger-Defiance and Low Task Orientation, though highly correlated, were found to be discriminable dimensions of children's functioning and to generate differential predictions regarding longitudinal persistence of emotional impairment.

The cross-syndrome correlations were not trivially small as expected but they were consistently lower than the same-syndrome correlations. Three cross-syndrome correlations remained significant after partialing: Early Low Task Orientation was linked with later Apathy-Withdrawal in the shorter prediction period. The other two correlations were inverse relationships: (a) Cooperation-Compliance, the healthy pole of the Anger-Defiance dimension, was associated with later Apathy-Withdrawal in both prediction periods. Thus, there appear to be two determinants of later Apathy-Withdrawal, early Apathy-Withdrawal and early Cooperation-Compliance. This finding is suggestive of the work of Stabenau and Pollin (1970) who identified inhibited as well as conforming behavior in the early personality patterns of children who in later life became schizophrenic.

(b) Interest-Participation, the healthy end of the Apathy-Withdrawal dimension, predicted to later Anger-Defiance in the within-elementary school period, indicating that both assertive and angry-defiant functioning seem to be antecedents of acting-out behavior.

All three correlations are explicable in terms of a circumplex model of social-emotional functioning (Emmerich, 1977; Schaefer, 1961, 1971) which will be discussed in chapter 10.

A comparison of the long-term and short-term predictions showed a general pattern of somewhat stronger relationships between predictor and criterion variables during the within-elementary school period than for the period, from preschool through fourth grade. The finding conformed to expectations. First of all, the longer time span represented a more extreme test of the longitudinal persistence hypothesis; second, the longer period involved a change in setting and the use of different instruments as the children moved from day care to elementary school; and third, stability of personality functioning probably increased with age.

An interesting exception to the general pattern involves the Apathy-Withdrawal syndrome. Correlations between the early syndrome scores and the later global ratings were larger when the time span between predictions was shorter in all instances but one: For Apathy-Withdrawal, correlations with Global Impairment were larger when preschool was the point of prediction. A similar finding was made in the grade-by-grade analysis reported in chapter 6 (see Table 6.6) where it was noted that teachers of young children appear to take inhibited functioning as more indicative of pathology than acting-out behavior. In contrast, elementary school teachers are more likely to consider acting-out behavior symptomatic of disturbance.

When persistence of emotional impairment was examined at successive age levels, results paralleling those summarized above were obtained. The syndromes remained moderately stable over time; after a lapse of four years between ratings, r values were still of respectable size. The cross-syndrome correlations were reduced markedly in longitudinal perspective. There was greater stability of functioning from one grade to another in elementary school, as the children grew older, than from preschool to first grade.

Anger-Defiance and Low Task Orientation, the acting-out syndromes, showed stronger longitudinal persistence than Apathy-Withdrawal, particularly when the children were very young. In later years the Apathy-Withdrawal scores tended to become more constant though still not as stable as those of the other dimensions. Schaefer (1975) has reported a similar finding.

All in all, our results supported neither the position that emotional problems in childhood are always transitory nor the viewpoint that early signs of disturbance are always premonitory. On the basis of the data analyses described in this chapter, we conclude that if a child shows a particular type of impairment at one age, there is a moderate probability that he will exhibit the same impairment at a later stage in his development.

As was pointed out earlier, significant longitudinal correlations between two measures may be caused by a third variable which maintains social-emotional functioning at a given level. Demographic data which might have served this purpose were controlled for in the present study. But there may be other factors which stabilize social-emotional functioning in childhood for considerable spans of time. Prime examples are variables dealing with the parent-child relationship. It was beyond the scope of the present study to collect data in this area but research into the psychodynamics of intrafamily interaction patterns would be valuable in furthering our understanding both of the epidemiology and longitudinal persistence of emotional impairment.

* * *

To sum up, of the four major hypotheses regarding the epidemiology and longitudinal persistence of emotional impairment, the first—linking emotional impairment and disadvantaged status—was supported sparsely; the second—dealing with persistence of type of impairment—was supported moderately, with each early syndrome predicting uniquely to the corresponding later syndrome; the third—postulating a relationship between early and later emotional impairment even after the demographic variables have been controlled for—was confirmed fully; the fourth—stating that the two classes of variables, taken jointly, would have greater value in predicting persistence of disturbance than when the demographic variables were used alone—was also fully borne out.

CHAPTER 8
Detection of High and Low Risk Children

In this chapter we will pursue the issue of longitudinal persistence of emotional impairment and approach the matter in a way directly meaningful to the clinician or researcher interested in the child "at risk." The questions posed in the present chapter are: If children are in the *most disturbed* group on any of the three dimensions at one point in data collection, what is the likelihood that they will still be in the *most disturbed* group on subsequent rating occasions? Since the three dimensions of social-emotional functioning are bipolar, we can also ask: If children are in the *healthiest* group on one of the three syndromes, what is the probability of their remaining in the *healthiest* group as they grow older?

In addition, we will address ourselves to the issue of change in level of social-emotional functioning, specifically to these questions: To what extent are children who are severely impaired on any of the dimensions when they are very young no longer in the most disturbed group at a later age? And to what extent are youngsters who show emotional health early in life no longer among the healthiest at a later time?

It is an indication of the profession's interest in pathology that we have a term for individuals who are likely to be emotionally impaired at a later point in their life: We call these individuals "at risk." According to Garmezy (1974), a child is at risk "if there is a greater likelihood that he will develop a mental disorder than a randomly selected child from the same community" (pp. 16–17).

There is, however, no commonly-accepted term for individuals with a prognosis of health. We will call these children "low risk" in contrast to the "high risk" children to whom Garmezy's definition refers. By "low risk" we mean more than absence of disturbance but, in line with Jahoda's (1958) concept, "positive mental health."

Methodology

For the purpose of the present analysis, the distribution of scores on each of the two syndromes assessed during the preschool period was split into three segments, as follows:

1. The top 25% of the distribution were the most disturbed children, i.e., those who had the highest scores on Apathy-Withdrawal and on Anger-Defiance.

2. The next 50% of the distribution constituted a middle group of children of "average" health.

3. The remaining 25% of the distribution were the healthiest children, i.e., those who had the lowest scores on Apathy-Withdrawal and Anger-Defiance or, to put it positively, the highest scores on the opposite poles, Interest-Participation and Cooperation-Compliance, respectively.

The same procedure was followed for the scores obtained at each grade level in elementary school. During the elementary school period, the distribution of Task Orientation scores was similarly divided into three segments.

Since there are large and mostly significant sex differences on each of the three syndromes at practically every age level, the cells containing the extremely disturbed and extremely healthy children were composed of an equal number of boys and girls. To accomplish this, the boys were ranked from most to least disturbed, and the extreme cases were assigned to the appropriate cells; the same procedure was followed for the girls. We could have undertaken two analyses, separately by sex, but we decided against this method because we wanted to have a large sample, particularly for the cross-tabulations involving longer spans of time.

Next, we carried out a series of cross-tabulations. For each syndrome the data from the first four time periods (preschool, first, second, and third grade) were cross-tabulated against the data from the last four time periods (first, second, third, and fourth grade).

With the exception of Schaefer (1971), previous researchers have not drawn a distinction between Anger-Defiance and Low Task Orientation but have frequently treated items reflecting these two dimensions in an undifferentiated way. For example, Peterson's (1961) list of Conduct problems contained Anger-Defiance items such as "disobedience," "disruptiveness," and "boisterousness" as well as some Low Task Orientation items such as "restlessness," "hyperactivity," and "distractibility." Similarly, Rutter's (1970) "antisocial disorders" category included traits reflecting both behavior patterns.

To determine stability when items from the two syndromes are considered simultaneously, we pooled the Anger-Defiance and Low Task Orientation scores; the distribution of the combined scores was divided into the three groups of most disturbed, average, and healthiest children, and the same cross-tabulations were carried out as for each of the syndromes.[27]

Results

The cross-tabulations at the various age levels are presented in Table 8.1. Since we will emphasize data bearing on healthy as

[27] For Low Task Orientation and the pooled syndromes, cross-tabulations began with first grade data.

Table 8.1 Longitudinal Persistence and Remission on Syndrome Measures

Part A: Interest-Participation versus Apathy-Withdrawal

	Preschool		1st grade		2nd grade		3rd grade	
	Disturbed	Healthy	Disturbed	Healthy	Disturbed	Healthy	Disturbed	Healthy
First grade								
Disturbed	43%	13%						
Healthy	11%	31%						
		$N=775$ $\chi^2=62$ $p \leqslant .01$						
Second grade								
Disturbed	44%	14%	49%	8%				
Healthy	10%	36%	10%	39%				
		$N=856$ $\chi^2=72$ $p \leqslant .01$		$N=664$ $\chi^2=91$ $p \leqslant .01$				
Third grade								
Disturbed	44%	14%	45%	16%	47%	8%		
Healthy	9%	34%	7%	37%	11%	45%		
		$N=670$ $\chi^2=61$ $p \leqslant .01$		$N=484$ $\chi^2=50$ $p \leqslant .01$		$N=564$ $\chi^2=79$ $p \leqslant .01$		
Fourth grade								
Disturbed	35%	16%	51%	15%	43%	9%	54%	10%
Healthy	12%	33%	6%	40%	8%	45%	5%	45%
		$N=323$ $\chi^2=17$ $p \leqslant .01$		$N=265$ $\chi^2=33$ $p \leqslant .01$		$N=246$ $\chi^2=31$ $p \leqslant .01$		$N=289$ $\chi^2=64$ $p \leqslant .01$

184

Table 8.1 (cont'd.)

Part B: Cooperation-Compliance versus Anger-Defiance

	Preschool		1st grade		2nd grade		3rd grade	
	Disturbed	Healthy	Disturbed	Healthy	Disturbed	Healthy	Disturbed	Healthy
First grade Disturbed Healthy	50% 10%	7% 41% $N = 779$ $\chi^2 = 113$ $p \leqslant .01$						
Second grade Disturbed Healthy	45% 9%	10% 49% $N = 856$ $\chi^2 = 132$ $p \leqslant .01$	44% 5%	5% 54% $N = 664$ $\chi^2 = 144$ $p \leqslant .01$				
Third grade Disturbed Healthy	37% 10%	14% 43% $N = 670$ $\chi^2 = 56$ $p \leqslant .01$	43% 8%	8% 48% $N = 484$ $\chi^2 = 74$ $p \leqslant .01$	52% 3%	6% 57% $N = 564$ $\chi^2 = 154$ $p \leqslant .01$		
Fourth grade Disturbed Healthy	41% 14%	13% 46% $N = 323$ $\chi^2 = 36$ $p \leqslant .01$	48% 8%	8% 42% $N = 265$ $\chi^2 = 34$ $p \leqslant .01$	46% 8%	9% 47% $N = 264$ $\chi^2 = 31$ $p \leqslant .01$	50% 5%	5% 56% $N = 289$ $\chi^2 = 65$ $p \leqslant .01$

Table 8.1 *(cont'd.)*

Part C: High versus Low Task Orientation

	Preschool		1st grade		2nd grade		3rd grade	
	Disturbed	Healthy	Disturbed	Healthy	Disturbed	Healthy	Disturbed	Healthy
First grade Disturbed	—	—						
Healthy	—	—						
Second grade Disturbed	—	—	45%	7%				
Healthy	—	—	5%	55%				
			$N = 659$ $\chi^2 = 142$ $p \leqslant .01$					
Third grade Disturbed	—	—	44%	8%	47%	5%		
Healthy	—	—	9%	50%	7%	57%		
			$N = 478$ $\chi^2 = 69$ $p \leqslant .01$		$N = 561$ $\chi^2 = 131$ $p \leqslant .01$			
Fourth grade Disturbed	—	—	40%	10%	36%	6%	55%	4%
Healthy	—	—	10%	39%	12%	47%	4%	48%
			$N = 265$ $\chi^2 = 21$ $p \leqslant .01$		$N = 244$ $\chi^2 = 25$ $p \leqslant .01$		$N = 287$ $\chi^2 = 69$ $p \leqslant .01$	

Table 8.1 (cont'd.)

Part D: Cooperation-Compliance versus Anger-Defiance Pooled With High versus Low Task Orientation

	Preschool		1st grade		2nd grade		3rd grade	
	Disturbed	Healthy	Disturbed	Healthy	Disturbed	Healthy	Disturbed	Healthy
First grade								
Disturbed	—	—						
Healthy	—	—						
Second grade								
Disturbed	—	—	49%	5%				
Healthy	—	—	5%	56%				
			$N = 659$					
			$\chi^2 = 176$					
			$p \leqslant .01$					
Third grade								
Disturbed	—	—	43%	4%	51%	3%		
Healthy	—	—	11%	54%	5%	57%		
			$N = 478$		$N = 561$			
			$\chi^2 = 88$		$\chi^2 = 156$			
			$p \leqslant .01$		$p \leqslant .01$			
Fourth grade								
Disturbed	—	—	41%	6%	46%	4%	48%	2%
Healthy	—	—	7%	40%	15%	46%	4%	57%
			$N = 265$		$N = 244$		$N = 287$	
			$\chi^2 = 29$		$\chi^2 = 34$		$\chi^2 = 66$	
			$p \leqslant .01$		$p \leqslant .01$		$p \leqslant .01$	

Note.—Disturbed and Healthy refer to the most disturbed 25% and the healthiest 25% of the children in the distribution. Data for the remaining children are not shown in the table but were included in the chi-square analysis. Each chi-square is based on $df = 4$. Scores are standard scores.

well as disturbed functioning, we are using the full designation of each dimension rather than the shortened version adopted for the sake of convenience in reporting results up to this point (see chapter 3).

Data on Interest-Participation versus Apathy-Withdrawal appear in Part A of the table, on Cooperation-Compliance versus Anger-Defiance in Part B, on High versus Low Task Orientation in Part C, and the results of pooling the scores of the latter two dimensions are shown in Part D of Table 8.1.

To simplify the presentation, the percentages of the group of average health are not shown in the table but can be easily inferred. For example, looking at the preschool to first grade cross-tabulation of Interest-Participation versus Apathy-Withdrawal cases, it may be seen that of the children who were rated most disturbed in the preschool period, 43% were still in the most disturbed group in first grade, and 11% moved to the healthiest group in first grade. This means that the remaining 46% received average scores. Similarly, it may be seen that 31% of the youngsters in the healthiest group in preschool remained in the healthiest group in first grade whereas 13% were now severely disturbed. Therefore, 56% obtained average scores in first grade.

All cross-tabulations have chi-square values which are significant at the 1% level or better. In other words, the probability of detecting high risk and low risk youngsters on the basis of their level of functioning at an earlier point in their life was substantially better than chance.

Persistence of disturbance

Many analyses could have been carried out with the data in Table 8.1; however, three comparisons were of major interest to us: (a) comparison of the preschool rating with all subsequent ratings to determine how accurately severely impaired children could be identified on the basis of their preschool scores (data appear in the first vertical column); (b) comparison of all fourth grade percentages with each other to ascertain how adequately disturbed fourth grade children could be selected at various grade levels prior to fourth grade (data may be found in the bottom rows); and (c) comparison of data along the first diagonal to see whether accuracy of prediction increased or decreased as the children became older. The first two comparisons involved varying time intervals between an earlier and a later point in data collection; in the third, time lapse between measurements was held constant at one year.

In order to have a convenient summary score, we also computed the median rate of longitudinal persistence for all time periods covered in the data analysis. We will now turn to Table 8.1.

Extent to which high risk children could be detected in preschool. Between 35% and 44% of the children who were among the most disturbed on Apathy-Withdrawal in preschool showed syndrome persistence from one to four years later. On Anger-Defiance, percentages varied from 37% to 50%. Severely disturbed behavior on Low Task Orientation (on which data collection began in first grade) was predictive of impaired functioning at later grade levels for 40% to 45% of the children.

Extent to which emotionally impaired fourth graders could be identified during earlier years of school attendance. As might be expected, accuracy in predicting the fourth grade measurements increased as the time span between ratings decreased. Table 8.1 data, presented in graphic form in Figure 7, show that the pattern was evident on all three syndrome measures.

Stability of functioning at different age levels. When time lapse between ratings was held constant at one year, the percentage of "correct" identifications rose with age for children high on Apathy-Withdrawal: During the first one-year interval between ratings—from preschool to first grade—43% of high risk children remained in the high risk group; during the last one-year interval—from third grade to fourth grade—the figure climbed to 54%.

Similarly, predictive power improved for children low on Task Orientation as they grew older: From first to second grade, 45% remained severely impaired whereas from third to fourth grade, 56% remained disturbed.

However, in the case of Anger-Defiance, as many youngsters (50%) were severely impaired from preschool to first grade as from third grade to fourth grade.

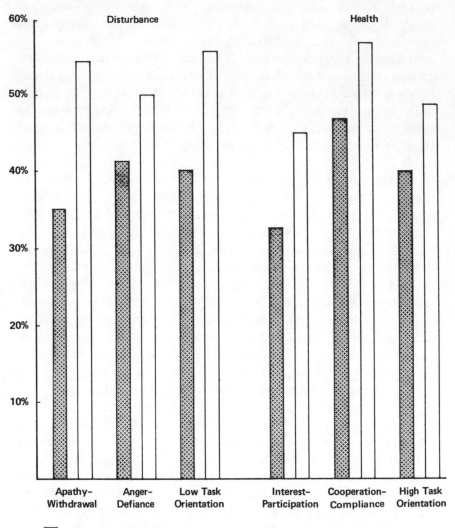

FIG. 7. Percentage of children remaining disturbed or healthy over a long as compared to a short prediction period.

Median rate of persistence. The median rate of persistence for all time periods covered in the data analysis was the same for all three syndromes—namely, 45%.

Effect of pooling Anger-Defiance and Low Task Orientation scores. On the whole, the gains from pooling the two syndromes were almost negligible. The initial rating was predictive for 41% to 49% of the disturbed children. Ability to detect impaired youngsters in fourth grade improved with shortened time intervals between ratings. Percentages along the first diagonal were remarkably constant as a result of combining the scores. The median persistence rate was 47%.

As indicated earlier, many researchers have treated these two facets of disturbed functioning in an undifferentiated way; however, considering them jointly does not appreciably enhance the likelihood of detecting high risk youngsters and only leads to loss of information.

Persistence of health

To determine persistence of healthy functioning, we carried out the same analyses reported for persistence of emotional impairment. In presenting data on the low risk children, however, we will depart from the practice of referring to the dimensions by the designation of the negative pole since the meaning of the results will be clearer and interpretation of the data facilitated if we use the label of the positive pole.

Extent to which low risk children could be detected in preschool. Between 31% and 36% of the youngsters who were among the healthiest on Interest-Participation during the preschool period maintained their level of functioning in the course of the next four years. On Cooperation-Compliance, between 41% and 49% remained in the low risk group in elementary school. First grade ratings of High Task Orientation were predictive of continued healthy functioning for 39% to 55% of the children.

Extent to which healthy fourth graders could be identified during earlier years of school attendance. In line with the findings on disturbance, on all three syndromes accuracy in selecting healthy fourth graders was inversely related to length of time span between ratings (see Figure 7).

Stability of functioning at different age levels. With one-year intervals between measurements, stability of healthy functioning increased with age on Interest-Participation (from 31%, preschool to first grade, to 45%, third grade to fourth grade) and on Cooperation-Compliance (from 41%, preschool to first grade, to 56%, third grade to fourth grade). The trend was not evident on High Task Orientation.

Median rate of persistence. The median rate of persistence of healthy functioning was 38% on Interest-Participation, 48% on Cooperation-Compliance, and 49% on High Task Orientation.

Effect of pooling Cooperation-Compliance and High Task Orientation scores. There were small gains as a consequence of pooling the scores of the two dimensions. Between 40% and 56% of the low risk children stayed in the healthiest group between the initial rating and subsequent measurements. Accuracy of predicting fourth grade functioning increased as time periods between ratings became shorter. Percentages along the first diagonal were stable. The median rate of persistence for all time periods was 55%.

Remission from disturbance

Since change in level of functioning is the converse of persistence, we will examine remission data more briefly than longitudinal persistence data. We will (a) compare the preschool rating with the fourth grade rating only; (b) look at all shorter time intervals between measurements together; and (c) report the median remission rate for all time periods covered in the data analysis.

Extent of remission between preschool and fourth grade. Over the four-year span—from preschool to fourth grade—65% of the children high on Apathy-Withdrawal[28] and 59% of the

[28] Remission data were calculated by subtracting the percentages shown in Table 8.1 from 100%. Thus, it may be seen in the first column in Part A of the table that 35% of the children remained severely disturbed from preschool to fourth grade. Consequently, 65% of the youngsters who were at high risk in preschool showed remission in fourth grade. And similarly, for the other syndromes.

youngsters high on Anger-Defiance recovered from emotional impairment; 60% of the children low on Task Orientation showed remission between first grade and fourth grade. The percentage of children moving from the most disturbed to the healthiest group was 12% on Apathy-Withdrawal, 14% on Anger-Defiance, and 10% on Low Task Orientation.

Extent of remission during all shorter time intervals between ratings. Remission rates ranged between 46% and 57% on Apathy-Withdrawal, 48% and 63% on Anger-Defiance, and 45% and 64% on Low Task Orientation. From 5% to 12% of the youngsters who were considered most severely disturbed at the initial point in data collection were rated among the healthiest in fourth grade.

Median rate of remission. The median rate of remission from disturbance on all three syndromes was 55%.

Effect of pooling Anger-Defiance and Low Task Orientation scores. By combining the scores of the two dimensions, the percentages changed only slightly. The median remission rate was 53%.

Remission from health

Webster's dictionary defines remission as "the act of remitting; a releasing, resigning, relinquishing." The term is usually applied to recovery from disturbance but the definition permits the term to be applied to a change from health to impairment, in the sense of relinquishing a state of well-being.

Our report will parallel the presentation on remission from disturbance, and we will use the designation of the positive poles of the dimensions in giving the results.

Extent of remission between preschool and fourth grade. The percentage of youngsters who were in the low risk group in preschool but were no longer rated among the healthiest four years later was 67% on Interest-Participation and 54% on Cooperation-Compliance. The remission rate on High Task Orientation between first grade and fourth grade was 61%. By fourth grade, 16% (Interest-Participation), 13% (Cooperation-Compliance), and 10% (High Task Orientation) were in fact exhibiting signs of disturbance.

Extent of remission during all shorter time intervals between ratings. From 55% to 69% of the children showed remission on Interest-Participation, 44% to 49% on Cooperation-Compliance, and 43% to 53% on High Task Orientation. The percentage of healthy children who were perceived severely disturbed on later rating occasions was lowest on High Task Orientation (4% to 8%) and highest on Interest-Participation (8% to 16%).

Median rate of remission. The median rate of remission from healthy functioning for all time periods was 62% on Interest-Participation, 52% on Cooperation-Compliance, and 51% on High Task Orientation.

Effect of pooling Cooperation-Compliance and High Task Orientation scores. The percentages changed to some extent when the two dimensions were pooled. The median remission rate was 45%.

Comparison of median rates of persistence and remission

For the sake of clarity of presentation, the median rates have been reported so far without special reference to the fact that for Interest-Participation versus Apathy-Withdrawal and Cooperation-Compliance versus Anger-Defiance, the median rates were averaged over all time periods beginning with preschool whereas for High versus Low Task Orientation and the pooled dimensions, the median rates were averaged over all time periods beginning with first grade.

To permit comparisons among all measures, we computed median rates excluding the preschool data. As shown in Table 8.2, the figures changed only slightly when the preschool data were removed. The median rate of persistence of disturbed functioning was still approximately the same on the three syndromes (ranging from 45% to 48%); pooling Anger-Defiance and Low Task Orientation did not produce an improvement over the rates of the constituent parts (47%).

Persistence of healthy functioning varied with the syndrome. The median rate was lowest on Interest-Participation (42%) and considerably higher on Cooperation-Compliance (51%) and High Task Orientation (49%). Combining the scores of the latter two resulted in a gain in the median rate (55%).

Table 8.2 Median Rates of Persistence and Remission

Syndromes	Persistence		Remission	
	Preschool data		Preschool data	
	With	Without	With	Without
Disturbance				
Apathy-Withdrawal	45%	48%	55%	52%
Anger-Defiance	45%	47%	55%	53%
Low Task Orientation		45%		55%
A-D and LTO pooled[a]		47%		53%
Health				
Interest-Participation	38%	42%	62%	58%
Cooperation-Compliance	48%	51%	52%	49%
High Task Orientation		49%		51%
C-C and HTO pooled[b]		55%		45%

[a] A-D and LTO pooled = Anger-Defiance and Low Task Orientation pooled.

[b] C-C and HTO pooled = Cooperation-Compliance and High Task Orientation pooled.

Remission data showed the converse pattern.

Comparing the healthy with the disturbed end of each syndrome, it is clear that Interest-Participation was less stable than its polar opposite, Apathy-Withdrawal. This result suggests that the generally lower longitudinal persistence correlations which were found for Interest-Participation versus Apathy-Withdrawal than for the other two dimensions of social-emotional functioning (see chapter 7) were primarily due to the lower stability of the healthy pole. On the other two syndromes, emotional well-being was slightly more enduring than emotional disturbance.

The greater longitudinal stability of Anger-Defiance has been ascribed to the fact that behavior which falls under the Anger-Defiance rubric has greater stimulus impact on the observer and is, therefore, assessed more reliably. This argument does not appear very plausible for two reasons. First, we have shown in chapter 3 that interrater reliability was as high for Apathy-Withdrawal as for Anger-Defiance. Second, this line of reasoning implies that the Cooperation-Compliance end of the

Cooperation-Compliance versus Anger-Defiance continuum would also be assessed less reliably since cooperative-compliant behavior is similar to apathetic-withdrawn behavior in being unspectacular. However, inspection of Part B of Table 8.1 reveals that, in eight out of ten cross-tabulations, the identification of cooperative-compliant children was in fact more accurate than identification of angry-defiant youngsters.

Stability and Independence of Factor Dimensions

We saw in chapter 7 (see Table 7.8) that the factor dimensions, when measured at the same point in time, were not completely independent of each other. It will be recalled that Apathy-Withdrawal was moderately correlated ($r = .35$) with Anger-Defiance during the preschool period. In elementary school the correlations between Apathy-Withdrawal and Anger-Defiance ranged from $r = .32$ to $r = .38$; the correlations between Apathy-Withdrawal and Low Task Orientation, from $r = .26$ to $r = .36$; and the correlations between Anger-Defiance and Low Task Orientation, from $r = .70$ to $r = .78$.

The magnitude of these correlations raises a question about the meaning of identifying high risk and low risk children: To the extent that there is a correlation between Apathy-Withdrawal and Anger-Defiance, when we are identifying children chronically impaired (or healthy) on one dimension, we may inadvertently be selecting children who will be chronically impaired (or healthy) on the other dimension. The problem is even bigger with respect to Anger-Defiance and Low Task Orientation: Because of the larger correlations between these two syndromes, the chances of considering a youngster chronically impaired on Anger-Defiance, when he is severely disturbed on Low Task Orientation, are greater.

However, we also noted in chapter 7 that the correlations between different syndromes were greatly attenuated over time. As the cross-syndrome correlations become smaller, the likelihood of considering a child chronically impaired on one syndrome when he is high on another syndrome is reduced. The probability approaches zero as cross-syndrome correlations approach zero over time.

The cross-syndrome correlations, shown in Table 7.8, have these implications for the detection of high and low risk children: When we select, on the basis of preschool or first grade data, a group of children who we think will be disturbed on the Apathy-Withdrawal dimension at a later time, we need not be concerned that there will be a greater-than-chance probability of identifying youngsters who will be impaired on Anger-Defiance or Low Task Orientation. Conversely, when we predict that a group of children will be high on Anger-Defiance or Low Task Orientation, we can rest assured that we are not confounding them with youngsters impaired on Apathy-Withdrawal. The same conclusions apply to children showing healthy functioning on these dimensions.

However, we cannot be as certain when we select children high on Anger-Defiance that we are not unwittingly picking out children low on Task Orientation. The more sizeable correlations between the acting-out syndromes imply that our chances of isolating children impaired on Anger-Defiance from those disturbed on Low Task Orientation are not very good. The same conclusion pertains to youngsters showing healthy functioning on these dimensions.

Conclusions

The questions posed at the beginning of the chapter can now be answered: There is a moderate likelihood that children who are among the most disturbed or among the healthiest on a particular dimension in the early years of life will remain disturbed or healthy on that syndrome at a later age.

However, while the persistence percentages were impressive (the median rate for all time intervals available on each of the syndromes was 45% on disturbed behavior and varied from 38% to 49% on healthy functioning), the figures showing change in level of social-emotional functioning were higher (i.e., the median rate for all available time periods was 55% on disturbance and ranged between 51% and 62% on healthy functioning). When the scores of two of the dimensions were pooled, the median rate of persistence was relatively unchanged on disturbance and showed a gain on health.

The data revealed a trend for persistence to decrease and remission to increase as the time span between rating occasions became longer.

In view of the considerable amount of remission, the question arises as to how seriously persistence data should be taken. The issue has both practical and theoretical aspects. Let us take the practical considerations first and make the following assumptions: (a) We want to conduct a therapeutic intervention program for children most likely to be seriously disturbed on the Anger-Defiance dimension two years from now; (b) we take a group of 100 youngsters in first grade; (c) the 25% cut-off point is valid; and (d) the 45% persistence rate applies to the two-year time lapse between measurements.

Without the screening process we would have to direct our interventional effort at the entire group in order to reach all of the youngsters who will be impaired; we would thus involve a very large number of children who did not require therapeutic intervention.

However, by focusing on the 25% with the highest scores on Anger-Defiance and knowing that almost half of this group will be severely impaired two years later, we will have cut drastically the proportion of children for whom treatment was not necessary. With sizeable groups of children, these early identification procedures can, therefore, result in considerable savings of effort and resources.

From a theoretical point of view, the answer depends on the time frame in which the reader is interested. For a comparatively short span of the life cycle, such as the years between preschool and the first four years of elementary school, persistence data should be taken seriously because our results suggest that a relatively large proportion of children both at high and low risk can be identified. However, as the prediction period becomes longer, the percentage of youngsters showing remission increases to the point where early detection is not feasible, at least with these procedures.

Even so, our results reveal considerably more stability than the findings reported by Shepherd et al. (1971). Using a measure based on total number of symptoms, they found that only 27% of children "deviant" in 1961 were still deviant three years later.

In our data the percentage of youngsters showing stable functioning after a four-year period did not go below 35%. Shepherd et al. pointed out that spontaneous remission was so widespread that only the rare child needed to enter treatment. There is no doubt that the amount of remission was large; however, a convincing argument can be made on behalf of the other side of the coin: that the percentage of children still disturbed after several years was impressive.

It is interesting to contrast the results on recovery reported in the present study as well as Shepherd et al.'s study, both of which used a randomly selected sample of normal children, with the findings of Robins (1966) whose investigation was described in chapter 2. Robins' sample consisted of adolescent psychiatric clinic patients. After a period of 30 years, only 16% of the patients referred for antisocial behavior and 30% of the cases classified as showing non-antisocial symptoms were diagnosed as psychiatrically well. While differences in methods and time element make comparisons among these various studies difficult, two points need to be emphasized:

1. It is plausible to find a lower rate of remission among individuals disturbed enough to be referred to a child guidance clinic.

2. As with most clinic cases, extensive interview data and other reports covering the children's behavior both in a variety of settings (home, school, and neighborhood) and over lengthy periods of time were gathered. Hence, the measures of emotional impairment were more broadly based and more stable than our elementary school data which consisted of ratings carried out once a year by a single teacher. Had our data been based on a number of evaluations made in a variety of settings, the longitudinal persistence of the traits under study would probably have been higher.

In a previous study (Kohn & Rosman, 1973b) we collected assessments of Interest-Participation versus Apathy-Withdrawal and Cooperation-Compliance versus Anger-Defiance in two behavior settings, a classroom and a test-taking situation, both in preschool and in elementary school. Longitudinal correlations ranged from .38 to .43 when a difference in setting was introduced. When the ratings from the two settings were pooled, both dimensions showed considerable gain in longitudinal persistence ($r = .60$ and $r = .65$, respectively, both $p \leqslant .01$).

As we will suggest in chapter 10, the accuracy of early detection can probably be enhanced by taking into account family variables, such as parental disturbance, psychopathology of siblings, etc., as well as constitutional/genetic factors which are predictive of risk in index cases.

The present findings raise provocative questions for the clinical investigator: Why do some children remain disturbed while others recover and are able to function with personal strength and adequacy in the classroom? What roots in the biological make-up or social environment lead to prolonged as compared to temporary impairment? And similarly with healthy youngsters, why do some stay healthy while others develop difficulties or even become seriously disturbed? Our results indicate that it is technically feasible to pursue these questions in further research.

CHAPTER 9
Relationship between Emotional Impairment and Academic Underachievement

In recent years there has been a great deal of justified concern with the poor school achievement of lower-class and minority-group children. Research has shown that these children have deficits in cognitive functioning which antedate the beginning of formal education, and a major strategy of the "war on poverty" in the 1960's was to implement nationwide intervention programs such as "Head Start" to prevent or remediate early cognitive deficits.

The preoccupation with preschool cognitive deficits as one of the major reasons for underachievement in elementary school has almost blinded early childhood psychologists and educators to other approaches; specifically, formulations about the relationship between emotional impairment and academic performance have been overlooked.

Since the early days of psychoanalysis the consensus of clinical thinking has been that learning difficulties were intimately related to the vicissitudes of the child's social and emotional development and to the nature of the resolution of conflicts (see Freud, A., 1931; Freud, S., 1933; Katan, 1961; Pearson, 1952). As Ekstein and Motto (1969) stated: "Through most of the history of psychoanalysis we find bridges which lead from the area of psychoanalysis to the area of education. There has always been a strong relationship between these two endeavors, although a changing one" (p. 3).

Psychoanalytic theory of personality functioning and development is very complex, and it was Freud's theoretical position that no symptom was fully understood unless genetic, structural, and psychodynamic factors were taken into account. *Post hoc* explanations of a variety of learning problems have been made by drawing on all of these facets, sometimes emphasizing one and sometimes another feature of the theory (see Pearson, 1952). What is lacking is a coherent framework of testable hypotheses.

Empirical research by a number of investigators (Bower, 1969; Harris, 1961; Olson, 1930; Stennett, 1966) has provided support for the assumption that there is a connection between emotional impairment and underachievement. But, as noted in chapter 1, in school-age children, causal inferences are not easily drawn: It is generally assumed that pathology leads to underachievement; however, the cause-effect relationship may flow in the opposite direction, and failure to achieve may result in emotional impairment. Moreover, these studies relied primarily on global and one-dimensional measures of disturbance.

Where differentiated measures were used with preadolescents and adolescents (see President's Commission on Law Enforcement and Administration of Justice, 1967; Rutter et al., 1970), underachievement has generally been associated with antisocial behavior (Anger-Defiance), but little evidence has been presented as to the age level at which the relationship first appears. Emmerich (1977) and Richards and McCandless (1972) reported that in young children Apathy-Withdrawal and not Anger-Defiance was related to underachievement.

In two previous studies conducted in this laboratory, cognition deficits and low academic attainment were also found to be linked to apathetic-withdrawn rather than angry-defiant behavior. In the study designed to determine the effectiveness of a program of therapeutic intervention with emotionally disturbed children in day care (see chapter 3), we examined, through an adaptation of the Rorschach test, the extent of stereotyped as compared to non-stereotyped thinking in children, ages 3 to 5. There was a direct relationship ($r = .35$, $p \leqslant .01$) between stereotyped thinking and Apathy-Withdrawal (Kohn, 1968).

In the second study, which was designed to investigate in a more comprehensive way the relationship between social-emotional and cognitive functioning (Kohn & Rosman, 1973a), we found that 5-year-old boys high on Apathy-Withdrawal did more poorly than boys high on Interest-Participation both on measures which capitalize on previous learning, such as the Caldwell Preschool Inventory (Caldwell, 1967), and on tasks which make minimal use of previous learning but require active mental processes, such as Raven's Progressive Matrices (Raven, 1956). Anger-Defiance was relatively unrelated to these indices of cognitive functioning.

In the present study we also assessed social-emotional functioning before the child began his formal education and, therefore, were in a position to test whether emotional difficulties existing prior to entry into elementary school were related to academic deficiencies in subsequent years. In addition, we expected to determine which syndrome was more closely related to and predictive of underachievement. Although our major interest was in the relationship between emotional impairment and underachievement, we were also concerned with the effect of demographic factors on some of the achievement variables.

Major Hypotheses

The major hypotheses were that:

1. The sociocultural matrix in which the child is embedded affects his school achievement; specifically, underachievement is a function of disadvantaged status.

2. Early emotional impairment is predictive of later underachievement; however, not all types of impairment are related equally to scholastic performance: Some syndromes are strongly related whereas others are minimally related.

3. Early emotional impairment is predictive of later underachievement over and above the demographic variables, i.e., after the demographic variables have been removed as a source of variability.

4. When demographic variables and early emotional impairment are taken jointly to predict academic attainment, the magnitude of the relationship will be greater than when the demographic variables are used alone.

More specific hypotheses will be spelled out later in the chapter.

Methods of Data Analysis

The study of the relationship between emotional impairment and academic underachievement paralleled in many ways the investigation into the epidemiology and longitudinal persistence of emotional impairment (see chapter 7).

The principal classes of variables—demographic data relevant to disadvantaged status and measures of emotional impairment—were the same. The same methods of data analysis—correlational and hierarchical multiple regression techniques—were used. To avoid repetitiousness and prohibitive costs, it was again necessary to select from a very large number of possible hierarchical multiple regression equations involving each of the grade levels in turn the particular ones which would yield the most vital and meaningful data with which to test the hypotheses.

We decided that two prediction periods would be especially instructive: (a) from preschool to third grade. For this period, predictions were made from the child's social-emotional functioning in day care (averaged over all rating occasions) to Verbal and Arithmetic Achievement in third grade. We would have liked to use fourth grade data as the criterion variables since these would have provided a more severe test of the hypotheses. However, since the arithmetic subtests of the

Metropolitan Achievement Tests are administered in grade 3 (not again until grade 6) and since we wished to make comparable analyses for Verbal and Arithmetic Achievement, we decided to use third grade variables as the outcome measures.

(b) From early elementary school to third grade. For this period, predictions were made from the child's social-emotional functioning (grades 1 and 2 averaged) to third grade (for reasons stated above).

Our principal interest was in the longer period because we were eager to learn whether emotional impairment related to underachievement antedated the onset of formal education. We performed the within-elementary school analysis for several reasons; primarily, to determine whether Low Task Orientation, which was not assessed during the preschool period, would have any predictive significance for intellectual functioning. As in chapter 7, the question was whether, in view of the high correlation between Anger-Defiance and Low Task Orientation, the two syndromes would relate differentially to the outcome measures. The fact that we had already found that each syndrome pattern, examined longitudinally, predicted uniquely to itself encouraged us to hold to the position that Low Task Orientation and Anger-Defiance would generate differential predictions to achievement.

We also wanted to determine to what extent the magnitude of the prediction would be enhanced (a) if the time span were shorter, and (b) when the social-emotional variables were assessed in the same setting where the child received his formal education. In addition, we wondered whether there would be a closer association between antisocial behavior (Anger-Defiance) and underachievement from a prediction point later than preschool.

Because of the cost involved, hierarchical multiple regression analyses were not carried out for Academic Standing and Grade Placement. Instead, two sets of correlation matrices were constructed, one relating preschool data and the other, first grade data, to second, third, and fourth grade scores on each of these criterion measures. The correlational technique was also used to examine Level Within Grade data which were obtained on the last rating occasion only.

The data analysis was divided into several parts; the methods, specific hypotheses, and findings will be presented in the next four sections of the chapter.

PART A: FROM PRESCHOOL TO THIRD GRADE

This analysis was carried out for Cohorts A and B.

Variables

Dependent variables

The two criterion measures were third grade Verbal Achievement and third grade Arithmetic Achievement. We were interested in comparing achievement in these two subject areas since it has frequently been asserted (see Bower, 1969) that in emotionally impaired children deficiencies in arithmetic are even more severe than deficiencies in reading.

Independent variables

The chief independent variables were the demographic data—age, sex, social class (as measured by mother's education), family intactness, and race-ethnicity—and the preschool emotional impairment measures—Apathy-Withdrawal, Anger-Defiance, Global Impairment, and Referral.

In addition, Verbal Fluency was used as a predictor variable and, for reasons to be explained presently, a separate procedural variable relating to the manner in which the achievement tests were administered was also utilized.

The independent variables were introduced into the multiple hierarchical regression equation in successive sets to determine the incremental variance contributed by each set. The sequential order of the sets and the hypotheses regarding the variables within each set are given below.

Definition of Sets and Related Hypotheses

Procedural variable set

Set 1: Test administration. Children attending the New York City public schools took the Metropolitan Achievement Tests in a group in their classrooms. Children enrolled in parochial or private schools were given the same tests on an individual basis by a member of the research staff. In order to control for the difference in circumstances under which the examinations were administered, a variable representing the testing procedure was introduced as the first set in the hierarchical multiple regression equation. (The data were coded: "individual" = 1; "group administration" = 2.)

In line with general findings, we expected the scores from the group tests to be lower than the scores from examinations administered in individualized testing sessions.

Demographic data sets

These sets were introduced in the same sequence as outlined in chapter 7 and for the same reasons—to avoid both spurious results and confounding effects.

Set 2: Demographic variables. The set included age at beginning of the study, sex, social class, and family intactness.

(a) Age. Since scores on achievement tests increase with age, we expected age to account for a modest amount of variance of the outcome measures.

(b) Sex. We predicted that girls would outperform boys, particularly in verbal facility.

Age and sex were analyzed in detail in chapter 6 and were entered here primarily to remove their effects before we exmained the other variables.

(c) Social class. The relationship of cognitive functioning and school achievement to social class has been one of the most consistent findings in the child development literature (Bayley, 1965). In accordance with past findings, we anticipated that social class would be predictive of both Verbal and Arithmetic Achievement and that achievement deficit would increase as social class level declined.

(d) Family intactness. There have been conflicting findings on the effect of broken family life on a child's intellectual functioning. Deutsch and Brown (1964) and Blanchard (1970) found that academic attainment of children from broken homes was lower than that of children from intact families. This result was not obtained in our investigations (Kohn & Cohen, 1975; Kohn & Rosman, 1972a, 1973a) nor in studies reported by Lurie (1970), Wasserman (1969), and Whiteman and Deutsch (1968). No prediction was made but the question was of particular interest since slightly more than half of the sample came from broken homes.

Set 3: Race and ethnic variables. There were two variables in this set. One was designed to compare white children with black and Puerto Rican children to determine the effect of minority-group status; the other compared black youngsters with Puerto Rican youngsters to ascertain differences between the two minority groups.

In line with findings about the detrimental influence of minority-group status on educational progress (Coleman, 1966; Deutsch & Associates, 1967) and speculations that differences in intellectual ability may be attributable to race (Jensen, 1968), we hypothesized that black and Puerto Rican children would show lower levels of academic achievement than white children. However, we assumed that the magnitude of the correlations would be sharply reduced after the variables frequently confounded with minority-group status, social class and family intactness, had been controlled for. Because of the language handicap, Puerto Rican children were expected to perform significantly more poorly than black children on the academic attainment measures.

Preschool emotional impairment sets

Set 4: Syndrome variables. Apathy-Withdrawal and Anger-Defiance constituted the variables in this set. We predicted that both syndromes would be related to underachievement. Because of previous findings cited at the beginning of the chapter, there was reason to expect a stronger association between Apathy-Withdrawal and underachievement when the children were very young and a stronger association between Anger-Defiance and underachievement at older age levels.

Set 5: Global variables. This set consisted of Global Impairment and Referral. It was anticipated that the set would contribute only a trivial amount of variance to the prediction of achievement; we hypothesized significant 1:1 correlations between the global ratings and intellectual achievement but after controlling for the syndrome variables, we expected the magnitude of the correlations to become negligible.

Verbal Fluency Set

Set 6: Verbal Fluency. We were interested in determining to what extent a measure of intellectual ability would be predictive of achievement over and above the demographic and emotional impairment variables. Moreover, there was the possibility that the teachers' ratings of a child's social-emotional functioning were in fact assessments of the child's intelligence. By introducing Verbal Fluency after the emotional impairment measures into the regression equation, we were able to put this question to a test. If the teachers' ratings of social-emotional functioning actually measured cognitive functioning. Verbal Fluency would lose predictive value after the emotional impairment variables had been partialed out.

Results

The findings are presented in Table 9.1 For each set, the incremental variance ($\Delta R^2 \%$) contributed by the set and level of significance are shown. Then the zero-order correlations (r_o) and the partial correlations (r_p) are given. The final lines of the table show the total amount of variance accounted for by all sets (total $R^2 \%$) and the corresponding multiple R value as well as the corrected $R^2 \%$ and corrected R (see McNemar, 1969).

Relationship between predictor variables and achievement measures

Set 1: Test administration. This variable accounted for a significant amount of variance of Verbal Achievement (2.3%) and of Arithmetic Achievement (4.8%). As expected, scores on group-administered tests were significantly lower than scores on individually-administered tests on both measures ($r = -.15$ for Verbal Achievement and $r = -.22$ for Arithmetic Achievement, both $p \leqslant .001$).

Table 9.1 Relationship between Demographic and Preschool Social-Emotional Variables and Third Grade Achievement Measures

Demographic & Preschool social-emotional variables	Metropolitan Achievement Tests							
	Verbal Achievement				Arithmetic Achievement			
	df	$\Delta R^2\%$	r_o	r_p	df	$\Delta R^2\%$	r_o	r_p
Set 1								
Test administration	1/640	2.3***	−.15***	−.15***	1/515	4.8***	−.22***	−.22***
Set 2	4/636	8.0***			4/511	4.7***		
Age			.01	.01			.08	.09*
Sex			.12**	.11**			.02	.01
Social class			.26***	.25***			.17***	.16***
Family intactness			.07	.02			.12**	.11**
Set 3	2/634	2.7***			2/509	1.9**		
White versus Others			.16***	.17***			.14**	.14**
Black versus Puerto Rican			.08*	.08*			.03	.04
Set 4	2/632	6.6***			2/507	11.2***		
Preschool Apathy-Withdrawal			−.30***	−.22***			−.31***	−.23***
Preschool Anger-Defiance			−.19***	−.10*			−.25***	−.20***
Set 5	2/630	0.7			2/505	2.2***		
Preschool Global Impairment			−.30***	−.08			−.36***	−.13**
Preschool Referral			−.19***	.02			−.24***	−.07
Set 6	1/629	4.7***			1/504	5.9***		
Preschool Verbal Fluency			−.38***	−.24***			−.40***	−.27***
Total $R^2\%$	12/629	25.0***			12/504	30.7***		
R		.50				.56		
Corrected $R^2\%$		23.8				29.4		
Corrected R		.49				.54		

Note.—$\Delta R^2\% = (\Delta R \times 100)$ which shows the increment in variance contributed by each set; r_o = zero-order correlation; r_p = partial correlation.

Direction of scores is as follows: for demographic variables, a high score = female, high social class, broken home, white (in white versus others), black (in black versus Puerto Rican); for social-emotional variables, a high score = disturbance on all measures; for achievement variables, a high score = high achievement.

*$p < .05$.

**$p < .01$.

***$p < .001$.

Set 2: Demographic variables. The variables in set 2 collectively accounted for 8.0% of the variance of Verbal Achievement and 4.7% of the variance of Arithmetic Achievement. Verbal but not Arithmetic Achievement was significantly related to sex, with girls outperforming boys, as anticipated.

In line with past findings and our own hypothesis, a significant relationship between social class and both achievement measures indicated that low social class level predicted to low academic attainment. Social class was the most potent of the demographic predictor variables.

Family intactness was significantly correlated with Arithmetic Achievement but not with Verbal Achievement. The direction of the relationship indicates that children from broken families obtained lower scores on the mathematics tests than children from intact homes.

Set 3: Race and ethnic variables. This set accounted for a small but significant proportion of variance of both achievement measures (Verbal, 2.7%, and Arithmetic, 1.9%). As predicted, black and Puerto Rican children preformed significantly more poorly than white children. However, contrary to expectation, the magnitude of the correlations was not reduced after social class and family intactness had been partialed out. The findings suggest that the academic achievement level of the black and Puerto Rican youngsters was a function of minority-group membership.

Puerto Rican children obtained significantly lower scores than black children on the verbal tests, as anticipated, but there was no significant difference between the two minority groups on the mathematical tests.

Set 4: Syndrome variables. The set accounted for a significant proportion of the variance of both criterion measures, 6.6% of Verbal Achievement and 11.2% of Arithmetic Achievement. At the zero-order level, both syndromes were significantly correlated with both achievement variables; the Apathy-Withdrawal correlations were larger than the Anger-Defiance correlations. After partialing, the relationship between Apathy-Withdrawal and both achievement criteria as well as between Anger-Defiance and Arithmetic Achievement, though reduced in magnitude, remained significant at the .001 level; the r_p between Anger-Defiance and Verbal Achievement was significant only at the .05 level.

Thus, as hypothesized, emotional impairment at the preschool level was predictive of underachievement in elementary school, with Apathy-Withdrawal a somewhat more potent predictor than Anger-Defiance.

Set 5: Global variables. The set accounted for a significant amount of variance of Arithmetic (2.2%) but not of Verbal Achievement. As anticipated, all zero-order correlations were significant but after partialing, only Gobal Impairment was significantly correlated with the outcome measures (at the .01 level with Arithmetic Achievement but only at the .05 level with Verbal Achievement). The results indicate that a child who was rated disturbed in day care was likely to have learning problems in later years.

The small amount of incremental variance and the decline in the size of the correlations after the syndromes had been controlled for corresponded to expectations.

Set 6: Verbal Fluency. This measure accounted for a significant amount of variance of both Verbal and Arithmetic Achievement (4.7% and 5.9%, respectively). The percentages are high considering that Verbal Fluency was introduced into the equation after 11 previous variables had been partialed out. Both zero-order and partial correlations were significant and of respectable size and indicate a direct relationship between low verbal skills in preschool and learning problems in later years. The data suggest that an estimate of intelligence, however roughly measured, can contribute significantly to the prediction of school achievement.

The fact that Verbal Fluency had predictive value after the emotional impairment variables had been controlled for showed that the teachers' ratings were assessments of social-emotional and not cognitive functioning.

Total variance. The 12 predictor variables jointly accounted for 25.0% of the variability of Verbal Achievement and 30.7% of the variability of Arithmetic Achievement. These percentages are not large enough to permit predictions for individual children but they are sufficient for identifying groups of preschoolers who, on the basis of background and level of disturbance, are at risk with respect to underachievement.

Summary

Procedural variable. The difference in testing procedure accounted for small-to-modest but significant amounts of the variance of the criterion measures, with scores on examinations administered in groups significantly lower than scores on tests given on an individual basis. The remaining data were examined with the effect of the difference in test setting controlled for.

Demographic variables. The principal findings were:

1. The two sets containing demographic data jointly accounted for 10.7% of the variance of Verbal Achievement and 6.6% of the variance of Arithmetic Achievement.

2. As expected, girls were significantly superior to boys in verbal skills; there was no sex difference on Arithmetic Achievement.

3. Social class was the most potent of the demographic variables. As anticipated, children from lower-class families performed significantly more poorly on both criterion measures than children from families higher on the social scale.

4. Youngsters from broken families obtained lower scores on the math tests than children from intact homes; the variable was unrelated to Verbal Achievement.

5. The data supported the hypothesis that minority-group children would show lower levels of achievement than white children. Contrary to expectation, however, the magnitude of the correlations was not reduced after social class and family intactness had been partialed out, implying that the school performance of these youngsters was a reflection of the effects of minority-group status.

Black children outperformed Puerto Rican pupils on the verbal tests but not on the arithmetic tests.

Emotional impairment variables. The principal findings were:

1. As postulated, preschool emotional impairment was predictive of later underachievement; the preschool social-emotional measures had predictive power after the demographic

variables had been statistically controlled for. They contributed 7.3% to the variance of Verbal Achievement (as compared to 10.7% contributed by the demographic variables) and added 13.4% to the variance of Arithmetic Achievement (as compared to 6.6% contributed by the demographic variables).

2. In line with past findings, emotional impairment was more closely associated with poor performance in arithmetic than inability to achieve on verbal tasks and tests.

3. Children who were rated high on Apathy-Withdrawal during the preschool period performed poorly on both achievement criteria in elementary school, as anticipated. Contrary to expectation, preschool Anger-Defiance was also significantly correlated with Arithmetic Achievement ($p \leqslant .001$) and, to a lesser extent, with Verbal Achievement ($p \leqslant .05$).

4. The data confirmed the hypothesis that, with the syndromes controlled for, the global ratings would contribute only a trivial amount of variance to the prediction of school achievement. After partialing, only Global Impairment predicted to academic deficiencies in elementary school.

Verbal Fluency. This variable, conceived to be a rough measure of intelligence, was found to be directly related to both achievement criteria.

Joint effect of all variables. The 12 predictor variables together accounted for a large proportion of the variance of the outcome measures: 25.0% of the variance of Verbal Achievement and 30.7% of the variance of Arithmetic Achievement. The percentages are large enough to permit identification of groups of preschool children who are at risk of underachievement in elementary school.

PART B: WITHIN-ELEMENTARY SCHOOL

Data for Cohorts A and B were used in this analysis.

The dependent variables were third grade Verbal Achievement and third grade Arithmetic Achievement. The independent variables were test administration, the demographic data, and the elementary school measures of emotional impairment—Apathy-Withdrawal, Anger-Defiance, Low Task Orientation, Global Impairment, and Referral. For each of these measures, the first and second grade scores were averaged. Verbal Fluency unfortunately had to be omitted from this analysis because of incomplete data (Cohort A was not rated on this measure in first grade).

The sets were identical to those used in the preschool to third grade analysis except that Low Task Orientation was added to set 4; the sets were introduced into the regression equation in the same sequence as described in the preceding section of the chapter. The hypotheses regarding the variables within each set were unchanged; Low Task Orientation was expected to be related to underachievement.

Results

Relationship between predictor variables and achievement measures

Data are presented in Table 9.2. Due to a slightly different sample base, the findings for set 1 (test administration) varied very slightly from the results obtained in the preschool to third grade analysis. The findings for set 2 (demographic variables) and set 3 (race and ethnic variables) were the same as those reported in the preceding section of the chapter.

Set 4: Syndrome variables. This set accounted for a significant and relatively large proportion of the variance of both Verbal and Arithmetic Achievement (17.1% and 18.5%, respectively). The percentages were considerably higher than the amounts of variance contributed by the demographic data.

At the zero-order level, all correlations were significant. After partialing, Apathy-Withdrawal and Low Task Orientation remained significantly correlated ($p \leqslant .001$) with both criterion measures, indicating that impairment on these syndromes was predictive of poor academic performance. Anger-Defiance was no longer significantly related to Verbal Achievement but was significantly associated ($p \leqslant .05$) with Arithmetic Achievement. However, both the correlation with Verbal Achievement, which did not reach significance, and the correlation with Arithmetic Achievement, which did, underwent a change in direction. The data imply that, with the other two syndromes held constant,

Table 9.2 Relationship between Demographic and Early Elementary School Social-Emotional Variables and Third Grade Achievement Measures

Demographic & Early elementary school social-emotional variables	Metropolitan Achievement Tests							
	Verbal Achievement				Arithmetic Achievement			
	df	ΔR²%	r_o	r_p	df	ΔR²%	r_o	r_p
Set 1								
Test administration	1/609	2.1***	−.15***	−.15***	1/484	5.0***	−.23***	−.23***
Set 2	4/605	8.0***			4/480	4.7***		
Age			.01	.01			.08	.09*
Sex			.12**	.11**			.02	.01
Social class			.26***	.25***			.17***	.16***
Family intactness			.07	.02			.12**	.11**
Set 3	2/603	2.7***			2/478	1.9**		
White versus Others			.16***	.17***			.14**	.14**
Black versus Puerto Rican			.08*	.08*			.03	.04
Set 4	3/600	17.1***			3/475	18.5***		
Apathy-Withdrawal (1g & 2g)			−.30***	−.18***			−.30***	−.21***
Anger-Defiance (1g & 2g)			−.32***	.05			−.26***	.10*
Low Task Orientation (1g & 2g)			−.41***	−.28***			−.38***	−.31***
Set 5	2/598	1.9***			2/473	2.1***		
Global Impairment (1g & 2g)			−.41***	−.15***			−.38***	−.16***
Referral (1g & 2g)			−.32***	.01			−.30***	.04
Total R²%	12/598	31.8***			12/473	32.0***		
R		.57				.57		
Corrected R²%		30.4				30.6		
Corrected R		.55				.55		

Note.—ΔR²% = (ΔR × 100) which shows the increment in variance contributed by each set; r_o = zero-order correlation; r_p = partial correlation.

Direction of scores is as follows: for demographic variables, a high score = female, high social class, broken home, white (in white versus others), black (in black versus Puerto Rican); for all measures of social-emotional functioning, a high score = disturbance; for achievement variables, a high score = high achievement.

1g & 2g = scores from the two grade levels were averaged.

*p ≤ .05.
**p ≤ .01.
***p ≤ .001.

Table 9.3 Early Elementary School Syndrome Measures and Third Grade Achievement Variables: An Alternative Analysis

Syndrome measures	Metropolitan Achievement Tests					
	Verbal Achievement			Arithmetic Achievement		
	df	$\Delta R^2\%$	r_p	df	$\Delta R^2\%$	r_p
Set 4a	2/601	11.1***		2/476	10.7***	
Apathy-Withdrawal (1g & 2g)			−.18***			−.21***
Anger-Defiance (1g & 2g)			−.23***			−.18***
Set 4b	1/600	6.0***		1/475	7.8***	
Low Task Orientation (1g & 2g)			−.28***			−.31***

Note.−$\Delta R^2\%$ = (ΔR × 100) which shows the increment in variance contributed by each set; r_p = partial correlation.
High scores indicate disturbance and high achievement.
1g & 2g = scores from the two grade levels were averaged.
***$p \leqslant .001$.

the child who was rated cooperative-compliant (the healthy pole of the Anger-Defiance dimension) toward the beginning of his school career was potentially an underachiever.

Let us digress briefly to describe an alternative analysis which demonstrates the effect and importance of the partialing procedure. We divided the three variables in set 4 into two sets; set 4a contained the Apathy-Withdrawal and Anger-Defiance scores and set 4b, the Low Task Orientation scores. As may be seen in Table 9.3, the partial correlations between Anger-Defiance and both outcome measures remained significant at the .001 level. These results, like the zero-order correlations pattern, suggest that impairment on each syndrome was predictive of underachievement and roughly to the same degree. In other words, when the overlap between Anger-Defiance and Low Task Orientation is not removed, a spurious finding regarding the relationship between angry-defiant behavior and academic attainment is obtained. Therefore, it is important to place the three syndrome measures into the same set in order to partial them out from one another.

It will be recalled that data presented in chapter 7 showed that the three syndromes generated differential predictions regarding longitudinal persistence of emotional impairment, with each syndrome predicting uniquely to itself, and that although Anger-Defiance and Low Task Orientation were highly correlated, they represented different facets of disturbed functioning. Data in Table 9.2 indicate that when these two unique elements were examined for their relationship to underachievement, only Low Task Orientation turned out to be associated with poor school performance. The findings in fact suggest that Anger-Defiance and underachievement were related inversely.

Set 5: Global variables. The last set accounted for a small but significant amount (approximately 2%) of the variance of both dependent variables. All r_o values were significant, thus linking disturbed functioning and referral for treatment to low level of school achievement. After partialing, only Global Impairment was still significantly related to the achievement criteria but the correlations had shrunk considerably.

The results were in line with our assumption that the global ratings would contribute very little to the prediction equation after the syndrome measures had been partialed out.

Total variance. The 12 predictor variables jointly accounted for 31.8% of the variance of Verbal Achievement and 32.0% of the variance of Arithmetic Achievement. These amounts are not large enough to make predictions for individual children but are large enough to identify groups of youngsters likely to be deficient in verbal and mathematical skills.

Summary

The principal findings were:

1. Data on the difference in test setting were virtually unchanged from results obtained in the preschool to third grade analysis. The effects of the demographic variables were exactly the same as those reported previously.

2. The two sets containing the social-emotional measures jointly accounted for 19.0% of the variance of Verbal Achievement (or almost twice as much as the demographic data) and 20.6% of the variance of Arithmetic Achievement (or more than three times as much as the demographic data).

3. Apathy-Withdrawal and Low Task Orientation were predictive of underachievement on both criterion measures, as hypothesized. An inverse correlation between Anger-Defiance and Arithmetic Achievement suggested that behavior rated as

cooperative and compliant toward the beginning of elementary school was associated, to a small but significant extent, with poor performance in arithmetic in third grade.

4. Consistent with expectations, the global ratings accounted for only small amounts of incremental variance of the dependent variables. After partialing, Global Impairment remained significantly correlated with both achievement criteria.

5. The 12 independent variables, taken jointly, accounted for a substantial portion (32%) of the variability both of Verbal and of Arithmetic Achievement; the figure is high enough to pinpoint groups of children who are likely to perform poorly in each subject area.

PART C: LINEAR AND CURVILINEAR RELATIONSHIPS BETWEEN SOCIAL-EMOTIONAL FUNCTIONING AND ACADEMIC ATTAINMENT

As noted in earlier chapters, the dimensions of social-emotional functioning covered the entire spectrum from health to disturbance. Since zero-order and partial correlations assume linearity of regression, the two data analyses reported so far demonstrated only the presence of linear relationships between two of the syndromes of emotional impairment and underachievement. This approach left open the question whether the entire range of social-emotional functioning contributed equally to the variance of the achievement measures. It might be, e.g., that while disturbed children had difficulty mastering academic subjects, healthy children did not enjoy an advantage in learning efficiency.

To investigate this issue, we examined the relationship between Verbal Achievement and Arithmetic Achievement and the linear and curvilinear (quadratic) components of Interest-Participation versus Apathy-Withdrawal and High versus Low Task Orientation. (We tested only the two dimensions for which significant linear relationships with the dependent variables had been found.) We assumed that if impairment and health both had an effect on academic attainment, the relationship between social-emotional and intellectual functioning would be linear, as illustrated by line A in Figure 8. If, on the other hand,

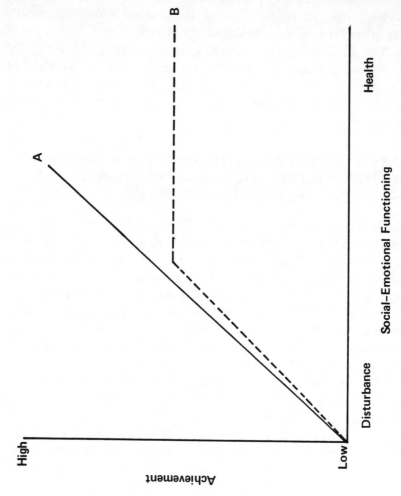

FIG. 8. Hypothetical linear and curvilinear relationships between social-emotional functioning and achievement.

disturbance was implicated in underachievement but health did not enhance chances of achievement, the relationship would be curvilinear, as shown graphically by line B in Figure 8. In the following analysis the linear and curvilinear (quadratic) components were partialed out from each other.

Results

The results of the analysis appear in Table 9.4, separately by sex. Part A of the table shows the linear and curvilinear correlations between the two dimensions and Verbal Achievement, and Part B shows comparable data for Arithmetic Achievement.

Interest-Participation versus Apathy-Withdrawal

All partial correlations of the linear relationship with the two criterion measures were highly significant ($p \leqslant .001$) for both sexes. On the other hand, only one of eight r_p values testing the curvilinear component was significant—namely, the partial correlation between the preschool score and Arithmetic Achievement for boys ($p \leqslant .05$).

These results clearly indicate that the disturbed child performed poorly on the cognitive tests while the healthy child obtained above average scores.

High versus Low Task Orientation

The partial correlations of the linear relationship with the achievement variables were all highly significant ($p \leqslant .001$) for boys and girls. For boys, the partial correlations measuring the curvilinear component were also significant ($p \leqslant .01$). In all likelihood, these r_p values are attributable to the fact that the scattergram (not shown) indicates that the achievement curve accelerated toward the High Task Orientation pole, suggesting that the more task-involved boys achieved at an exceptionally high rate.

Summary

The results suggest that the entire range of social-emotional functioning was implicated in school achievement. The pattern

Table 9.4 Linear and Curvilinear Relationships of Interest-Participation versus Apathy-Withdrawal and High versus Low Task Orientation to Verbal and Arithmetic Achievement

Syndrome measures	Boys			Girls		
	df	r_o	r_p	df	r_o	r_p
Part A: Verbal Achievement						
Interest-Participation versus Apathy-Withdrawal (preschool)						
Linear	1/345	−.30***	−.27***	1/339	−.23***	−.23***
Curvilinear	1/345	−	.03	1/339	−	.07
Interest-Participation versus Apathy-Withdrawal (1g & 2g)						
Linear	1/331	−.28***	−.18***	1/314	−.30***	−.22***
Curvilinear	1/331	−	.01	1/314	−	.05
High versus Low Task Orientation (1g & 2g)						
Linear	1/331	−.35***	−.37***	1/314	−.29***	−.28***
Curvilinear	1/331	−	−.16**	1/314	−	.05
Part B: Arithmetic Achievement						
Interest-Participation versus Apathy-Withdrawal (preschool)						
Linear	1/266	−.35***	−.37***	1/285	−.24***	−.25***
Curvilinear	1/266	−	.15*	1/285	−	.09
Interest-Participation versus Apathy-Withdrawal (1g & 2g)						
Linear	1/251	−.27***	−.22***	1/260	−.32***	−.26***
Curvilinear	1/251	−	.06	1/260	−	.08
High versus Low Task Orientation (1g & 2g)						
Linear	1/251	−.36***	−.37***	1/260	−.28***	−.25***
Curvilinear	1/251	−	−.16**	1/260	−	.09

Note.—High scores indicate disturbance and high achievement.
1g & 2g = scores from the two grade levels were averaged.
   *$p \leqslant .05$.
  **$p \leqslant .01$.
 ***$p \leqslant .001$.

varied with syndrome and sex. In the relationship between Interest-Participation versus Apathy-Withdrawal and the achievement variables, the linear component was of far greater significance than the curvilinear component for both sexes. The same was true of the relationship between High versus Low Task Orientation and the achievement criteria for girls; for boys, both components were significant on each measure. We may generalize that emotional impairment was found to exert a detrimental and emotional health a favorable influence on learning ability.

PART D: PREDICTIONS TO ADDITIONAL ACADEMIC CRITERIA

We studied the relationship between the syndromes of emotional impairment and three additional criteria of school achievement—namely, Academic Standing, Grade Placement, and Level Within Grade. Data for all three Cohorts were included in the analysis. Because of limited funds, we had to forego hierarchical multiple regression procedures and used only zero-order and partial correlations in this investigation. Separate matrices were obtained for boys and girls. For the partial correlation analyses, the three syndrome measures were partialed out from one another.

Results

Predictions from preschool syndrome measures

The findings for Academic Standing and Grade Placement appear in Table 9.5, those for Level Within Grade in Part A of Table 9.6.

Academic Standing. It will be recalled that Academic Standing was indicative of the child's scholastic performance relative to that of the other children in the class. The zero-order correlations suggest that the child who received high scores on Apathy-Withdrawal in preschool performed at a significantly lower level in elementary school than the child who was rated high on the polar opposite, Interest-Participation; all correlations (six out of six) were statistically significant. Anger-Defiance was less consistently correlated with Academic Standing: There was a trend for children high on Anger-Defiance in preschool to underachieve in elementary school but only four of six r_o's were significant. No clear pattern of sex differences emerged.

When the two syndromes were partialed out from each other, only Apathy-Withdrawal was still significantly associated with Academic Standing; none of the Anger-Defiance r_p's were significant. For boys, the Apathy-Withdrawal correlations were fairly stable from second to fourth grade whereas for girls, the correlations increased with age.

Table 9.5 Correlations between Preschool Syndrome Measures and Academic Standing and Grade Placement

Preschool syndrome measures	Achievement criteria					
	Boys			Girls		
	Part A: Academic Standing[a]					
	Grade			Grade		
	to 2nd $N = 495$	to 3rd $N = 389$	to 4th $N = 194$	to 2nd $N = 473$	to 3rd $N = 374$	to 4th $N = 186$
Apathy-Withdrawal						
r_o	−.30***	−.32***	−.28***	−.21***	−.32***	−.41***
r_p	−.27***	−.29***	−.26***	−.18***	−.30***	−.39***
Anger-Defiance						
r_o	−.15***	−.15**	−.10	−.12**	−.13**	−.12
r_p	−.05	−.04	.01	−.05	−.02	−.02
	Part B: Grade Placement[b]					
	to 2nd $N = 477$	by 3rd $N = 359$	by 4th $N = 169$	by 2nd $N = 463$	by 3rd $N = 351$	by 4th $N = 171$
Apathy-Withdrawal						
r_o	−.18***	−.19***	−.30***	−.12**	−.23***	−.27***
r_p	−.15***	−.17***	−.27***	−.10*	−.21***	−.20**
Anger-Defiance						
r_o	−.12**	−.10	−.14	−.07	−.11*	−.25***
r_p	−.06	−.03	−.04	−.03	−.03	−.17*

Note.—Direction of scores is as follows: On social-emotional measures, high scores = disturbance; on achievement criteria, high scores = superior Academic Standing and Grade Placement ahead of age group.

[a] Scores were averaged over grade levels, with a new score added to the average each year.

[b] Scores are cumulative

*p ≤ .05.
**p ≤ .01.
***p ≤ .001.

Grade Placement. This score showed whether the child was in the correct grade for his age, had advanced beyond or fallen behind his age group. Based on the zero-order correlations shown in Table 9.5, Apathy-Withdrawal had significant predictive value at every grade level for both sexes. The Apathy-Withdrawal correlations were generally more robust and more consistently significant than the Anger-Defiance correlations. The size of the correlations was about the same for both sexes. After partialing, all Apathy-Withdrawal correlations remained significant; the Anger-Defiance r_p's were no longer significant, with one exception (fourth grade, for girls).

Table 9.6 Correlations between Syndrome Measures and Level Within Grade

Syndrome measures	Achievement measure	
	Boys	Girls
Part A: Preschool		
	$N = 456$	$N = 448$
Apathy-Withdrawal		
r_o	−.23***	−.21***
r_p	−.21***	−.19***
Anger-Defiance		
r_o	−.09*	−.09*
r_p	−.01	−.02
Part B: First grade		
	$N = 426$	$N = 412$
Apathy-Withdrawal		
r_o	−.23***	−.24***
r_p	−.20***	−.18***
Anger-Defiance		
r_o	−.17***	−.24***
r_p	.05	.01
Low Task Orientation		
r_o	−.26***	−.30***
r_p	−.19***	−.20***

Note.−High scores indicate disturbance and class which is more advanced than others at the same grade level.
*$p \leqslant .05$.
***$p \leqslant .001$.

The Apathy-Withdrawal correlations rose over time for both sexes. The trend may be due, in part, to the fact that children are at higher risk of failing the longer they are in school; thus, the measure is a cumulative one and by definition oscillates around a higher mean value from one age level to the next.

Level Within Grade. On this measure, the teacher indicated whether the class the child was attending was, relative to the other classes at the same grade level, "among the brightest" = 3, "middle" = 2, or "among the slowest" = 1. Data were collected on the last rating occasion only when Cohort A was in fourth grade, Cohort B in third grade, and Cohort C in second grade.

The zero-order correlations in Part A of Table 9.6 show that children with high scores on Apathy-Withdrawal in day care were more likely to be in a slow class in elementary school than children who were rated high on Interest-Participation. The same pattern applied to the Cooperation-Compliance versus Anger-Defiance dimension but at a lower level of significance. After partialing, only the Apathy-Withdrawal correlations remained significant. There were no sex differences.

Predictions from first grade syndrome measures

The correlations between the three syndrome measures and Academic Standing and Grade Placement are displayed in Table 9.7, separately for boys and girls; data for Level Within Grade may be found in Part B of Table 9.6.

Academic Standing. For both sexes, the zero-order correlations between the three syndromes and this measure were generally highly significant, indicating that disturbance was a handicap to intellectual functioning. The strongest relationship was between Low Task Orientation and Academic Standing; the correlations between Apathy-Withdrawal and Academic Standing ranked second in size.

After partialing the three syndromes from one another, Low Task Orientation remained the most potent predictor of academic performance for both sexes (r_p values for Low Task Orientation varied from $-.33$ to $-.41$, $p \leqslant .001$; for Apathy-Withdrawal, from $-.27$, $p \leqslant .01$ to $-.37$, $p \leqslant .001$). The Anger-Defiance correlations again underwent a change in direction (cf. within-elementary school analysis described earlier in the chapter); furthermore, three of the six positive correlations were statistically significant (the range was from .06, *n.s.* to .18, $p \leqslant .001$). These results provide further evidence that when the dimension, Cooperation-Compliance versus Anger-Defiance, is related to measures of academic functioning after the effect of the other syndromes has been removed, it is not

Table 9.7 Correlations between First Grade Syndrome Measures and Academic Standing and Grade Placement

First grade syndrome measures	Achievement criteria					
	Boys			Girls		
Part A: Academic Standing[a]						
	Grade			Grade		
	to 2nd $N = 374$	to 3rd $N = 263$	to 4th $N = 139$	to 2nd $N = 360$	to 3rd $N = 250$	to 4th $N = 138$
Apathy-Withdrawal						
r_o	−.39***	−.35***	−.34***	−.33***	−.38***	−.38***
r_p	−.32***	−.30***	−.27***	−.28***	−.33***	−.37***
Anger-Defiance						
r_o	−.24***	−.24***	−.28***	−.28***	−.27***	−.13
r_p	.18***	.16***	.11	.06	.10	.17*
Low Task Orientation						
r_o	−.46***	−.43***	−.48***	−.42***	−.44***	−.33***
r_p	−.41***	−.39***	−.40***	−.33***	−.36***	−.33***
Part B: Grade Placement[b]						
	Grade			Grade		
	by 2nd $N = 374$	by 3rd $N = 263$	by 4th $N = 139$	by 2nd $N = 360$	by 3rd $N = 250$	by 4th $N = 138$
Apath-Withdrawal						
r_o	−.16**	−.19**	−.29***	−.03	−.20**	−.28***
r_p	−.13*	−.18**	−.25**	−.01	−.15*	−.23**
Anger-Defiance						
r_o	−.08	−.04	−.15	−.11*	−.18**	−.28***
r_p	.07	.15*	.06	−.05	−.03	−.05
Low Task Orientation						
r_o	−.17***	−.18**	−.23***	−.11*	−.20**	−.35***
r_p	−.14**	−.21***	−.17*	−.05	−.11	−.23**

Note. − Direction of scores is as follows: On social-emotional measures, high scores = disturbance; on achievement criteria, high scores = superior Academic Standing and Grade Placement ahead of age group.
[a] Scores were averaged over grade levels, with a new score added to the average each year.
[b] Scores are cumulative.
*$p \leqslant .05$.
**$p \leqslant .01$.
***$p \leqslant .001$.

the angry-defiant but the cooperative-compliant children who are at risk of underachievement.

No marked age trends were evident in the data.

Grade Placement. Of the three syndromes, Low Task Orientation and Apathy-Withdrawal were most strongly associated with this measure, indicating that children who were disturbed on these syndromes were likely to fall behind. For boys, all r_o and r_p values were significant; for girls, three of the six correlations lost significance after partialing. The correlations increased with age for both sexes.

The correlations between Anger-Defiance and Grade Placement were smaller than those of the other two syndromes. For girls, correlations were significant at the zero-order level but not after the syndromes had been partialed out from one another. For boys, correlations were not significant at the zero-order level; a reversal of signs in the partial correlations (one of which reached significance) suggested that the cooperative-compliant boy was more likely to be kept back than the angry-defiant boy.

Level Within Grade. As may be seen in Part B of Table 9.6, all zero-order correlations were highly significant, implying that children who were rated emotionally disturbed were likely to be assigned to a slow class. When the syndromes were partialed out from one another, Apathy-Withdrawal and Low Task Orientation retained significant predictive value; Anger-Defiance r_p's underwent a change in direction but did not reach significance. Boys' and girls' correlations were about the same order of magnitude.

Summary

The principal findings were:

1. When preschool was the point of prediction, for both sexes, Apathy-Withdrawal but not Anger-Defiance was related to Academic Standing, Grade Placement, and Level Within Grade. The data showed that the more disturbed the child, the greater the likelihood that he (a) would be ranked in the bottom third of his class, (b) would have to repeat a grade, and (c) would be assigned to a slow class within his grade level.

There was a tendency for the association between Apathy-Withdrawal and Grade Placement to increase with age for both sexes and for the association between Apathy-Withdrawal and Academic Standing to increase with age for girls.

2. When first grade was the point of prediction, Low Task Orientation and Apathy-Withdrawal were potent and independent predictors of all three academic criteria. In general, boys and girls showed similar patterns. The relationship between

the syndromes and Grade Placement became stronger over time.

There were small-to-modest zero-order correlations between Anger-Defiance and the outcome measures but after the other two syndromes had been partialed out, there was a trend for reversal of signs, and some of the partial correlations were significant. The data suggest that for boys, compliant rather than disruptive behavior was predictive of learning problems and of failing in school.

CONCLUSIONS

Underachievement as a Function of Emotional Impairment

The association between disturbance and school performance was tested against five achievement criteria—two standardized test measures, a teacher rating of academic performance, and two other variables.

The multiple hierarchical regression procedure allowed us to assess the relationship between social-emotional functioning and scores on the achievement tests with the effects of test administration (group versus individual) and demographic status controlled for. In the preschool to third grade prediction period, the syndrome and global measures together accounted for modest-to-moderate amounts of the variance of Verbal Achievement (7.3%) and Arithmetic Achievement (13.4%); in the within-elementary school analysis, for relatively large proportions of the variance of Verbal Achievement (19.0%) and Arithmetic Achievement (20.6%). In other words, the magnitude of the predictions was enhanced substantially (a) when the time span between ratings was shorter, (b) when social-emotional and cognitive functioning were assessed in the same setting, and, most importantly, (c) when a third syndrome measure—Low Task Orientation—was added.

The significant empirical relationship between preschool emotional impairment and low level of achievement in elementary school indicates that disturbed functioning antedated the beginning of formal education. The finding rules out the possibility that emotional problems are *solely* a consequence of educational failure. However, two alternative possibilities deserve further research: (a) that a link between pathology and cognition deficit already exists in the preschool years (some evidence of this was found in previous studies; see Kohn, 1968; Kohn & Rosman, 1973a), and (b) that if a child consistently ⤴ achieves less than is expected of him and falls progressively further behind, he may become disturbed.

When preschool was the point of prediction, children with emotional problems experienced greater difficulties with arithmetic than with language tests; this pattern was less pronounced in the within-elementary school analysis.

As anticipated, the syndrome measures were differentially related to academic underachievement. In the preschool to third grade prediction period, after correlations had been corrected for overlap, shy and withdrawn behavior was a more potent predictor of learning difficulties than angry-defiant behavior. These results correspond to our own previous findings (Kohn, 1968; Kohn & Rosman, 1972a, 1973a) and to those of Emmerich (1977) and Richards and McCandless (1972).

In the within-elementary school analysis, after partialing, Apathy-Withdrawal and Low Task Orientation, but not Anger-Defiance, were significantly associated with poor intellectual functioning. In fact, there was indication of an inverse relationship—namely, that cooperative-compliant behavior (the opposite pole of the Anger-Defiance dimension) signaled potential underachievement. This trend has emerged in a number of independent studies (Kohn & Rosman, 1973a, 1974).

The data suggest that investigators linking antisocial behavior to school failure may either have obtained spurious results because their measures did not distinguish between Anger-Defiance and Low Task Orientation or Anger-Defiance may in fact become related to underachievement at later age levels.

A simpler analysis (only zero-order and partial correlations) involving the syndrome measures and the three other academic criteria also yielded evidence that Apathy-Withdrawal and Low Task Orientation were implicated in underachievement. Although the five outcome measures are no doubt correlated with each other, the fact that the social-emotional variables predicted to a wide range of related criteria is impressive.

How can we explain the relationship of Apathy-Withdrawal and Low Task Orientation to underachievement? We postulate that the syndromes affect cognitive functioning in two ways:

1. Outer behavior: contact with the environment. Sontag, Baker, and Nelson (1958) and Kagan, Sontag, Baker, and Nelson (1958) found that the general trait of activity, in the sense of active coping, initiative, assertiveness, and curiosity, facilitated the learning of responses that are measured in intelligence tests. They further found that emotional independence from peers and teachers, the ability to operate freely and constructively in a preschool setting, assertiveness, interest, and curiosity were predictive of subsequent IQ gain.

The items at the healthy end of the Interest-Participation versus Apathy-Withdrawal dimension cover similar traits. Thus, it is our theory that the child high on Interest-Participation learns from his environment because of his curiosity, assertiveness, and high rate of social interaction; the apathetic-withdrawn child is slow to gain knowledge and skills because he is less exposed to environmental stimuli and has a low rate of social interaction; he may even actively avoid contact with others.

Along similar lines, the task-involved child absorbs ideas because he is well-organized and systematic in his contacts with the world around him whereas the hyperactive and restless child is not long enough in touch with specific objects, events, and people to learn anything about their characteristics and interrelations.

2. Inner behavior: mental processes. According to Bruner, as quoted by Pines (1970), learning about the environment and coping with it involve mental activities such as intention, hypothesis formulation, hypothesis testing, feedback from outcome to preconception, etc. It seems plausible that the child who exhibits curiosity and assertiveness is mentally alert and engages actively in the type of thought processes postulated by Bruner. On the other hand, the child showing passive behavior is likely to be mentally inert, less inclined to try to make sense of what goes on around him, and indifferent about verifying his ideas; he may even avoid thinking.

The High Task Orientation child is likely to be well-organized and systematic in the way he thinks whereas the child whose behavior is disorganized, distracted, and restless is likely to engage in mental processes that share these characteristics.

The data showed that the linear relationships between the two syndromes and the achievement test measures were generally of greater significance than the curvilinear patterns, indicating that academic attainment is related to social-emotional functioning along the entire continuum from health to disturbance. Thus, not only is the apathetic-withdrawn or hyperactive child handicapped in learning and thinking but a child's disposition to participate enthusiastically in activities or to give his undivided attention to a task brings about a gain in intellectual functioning.

Underachievement as a Function of Disadvantaged Status

In both prediction periods, the demographic variables accounted for 10.7% and 6.6%, respectively, of the variance of the youngsters' performance on the standardized verbal and arithmetic test measures. These percentages were lower than the amount of variability contributed by the social-emotional measures, with one exception: At the preschool level, background data accounted for a somewhat larger proportion of the variance of Verbal Achievement than the emotional impairment variables.

The results corroborated the widely held and well-documented view that disadvantaged status is a handicap to academic success (Bayley, 1940, 1954; Bernstein, 1961; Coleman, 1966; Dave, 1963; Deutsch & Associates, 1967; Golden, Birns, Bridger, & Moss, 1971; Gray & Klaus, 1965; McClelland, 1961; Moles, 1965; Wolf, 1963; among others).

Of the three indicators of disadvantaged status, social class was the most potent predictor of school failure. Consistent with past findings, academic deficiencies increased as social class level declined.

Family intactness was the weakest of the three indices: Children from broken homes performed significantly more poorly in arithmetic than children from intact homes but there was no significant difference in verbal ability.

Unexpectedly, the racial and ethnic variables had a significant influence on level of achievement. Correlations were not large but were significant at the .01 level or better. A great deal of previous data on the relative school achivement of minority-group and white children have been difficult to interpret because it was not clearly established that minority-group status and no other background variable was the causal factor in low academic attainment. In the present study we assumed that after we had statistically controlled for the effects of social class and family intactness, differences in school performance between white and minority-group children would be sharply reduced. This, however, was not the case, and the findings point to the conclusion that minority-group status has a small but deleterious impact on academic progress over and above the other two variables.

However, the data cannot be interpreted to support the explanation advanced by Jensen (1968) that black children, in particular, are genetically less endowed than white children. We believe, in line with the theoretical arguments propounded by Gottesman (1968) in regard to intelligence, that school achievement has multiple determinants, and unless and until all relevant variables have been matched, no valid conclusion can be drawn about genetic factors. In the present study we controlled for only two variables, social class and family intactness; we did not control for such other pertinent factors as, e.g., the relevance of standardized achievement tests to black and Puerto Rican children, psychological reactions to the experience of belonging to a minority group, etc.

* * *

To sum up, of the four major hypotheses regarding the relationship between emotional impairment and academic underachievement, the first—associating academic deficiencies with disadvantaged status—was generally confirmed; the second—stating that early emotional impairment was predictive of later underachievement—was supported fully, with

Apathy-Withdrawal and Low Task Orientation, but not Anger-Defiance, strongly related to poor intellectual development; the third—postulating a relationship between early emotional impairment and later underachievement even after the demographic variables have been controlled for—was borne out fully; the fourth—expecting the two classes of variables, taken jointly, to have greater value in predicting academic attainment than when the demographic data were used alone—was also fully confirmed.

CHAPTER 10
Summary, Interpretation, and Conclusion

Some readers will have arrived at this point in the book after careful and thorough examination of each chapter. Others will have probed in detail selected aspects of the research but taken a less demanding route through other portions of this volume. We will now present a compact overview of the study; offer commentary on the two-factor model of social-emotional functioning; point to those special features of the methodology which can be of primary value in risk research, particularly the great potential offered by the model; and suggest lines of inquiry which will extend the approach and findings of the present study into new directions.

Retrospective View

The present study was ambitious in aim, broad in focus, and large in operational scope. The aim was to demonstrate the usefulness of the two-factor model of social-emotional functioning in clinical and mental health research. The two factors were bipolar and were called:

Factor I: Interest-Participation versus Apathy-Withdrawal
Factor II: Cooperation-Compliance versus Anger-Defiance

The healthy pole of Factor I denoted curiosity, assertiveness, involvement in classroom activities, and positive interpersonal relationships with peers; the disturbed pole of Factor I was characterized by shyness, passivity, and isolation from classroom activities and peers. The healthy end of Factor II indicated willingness to conform to the rules, regulations, and routines of the classroom and adhere to the teacher's requests and suggestions; the disturbed end of Factor II involved rebelliousness, disruption of classroom routines, and hostile interactions with the other children.

The study focused on three interrelated areas of investigation: (a) the epidemiology of emotional impairment and academic underachievement in childhood, with particular emphasis on the effect of disadvantaged status variables on mental health and academic progress; (b) the longitudinal persistence of emotional impairment, including the extent to which both poorly functioning and healthy children can be detected at an early age; and (c) the relationship between emotional impairment and academic underachievement, especially the extent to which type and severity of disturbance prior to school entry are predictive of scholastic performance during the middle years of childhood.

Operational scope

The subjects were a 20% random sample ($N = 1,232$) of all children attending 90 public day care centers located in four boroughs of the City of New York. The children were composed of three age groups (3-, 4-, and 5-year-olds) and were followed for a period of five years, i.e., until the oldest group completed fourth grade.

Data were collected (a) by means of teacher ratings of the youngsters' social-emotional functioning on two preschool instruments (Symptom Checklist and Social Competence Scale, developed in this laboratory) and two elementary school instruments (Problem Checklist, developed by Peterson [1961], and Classroom Behavior Inventory, devised by Schaefer et al. [1965]); (b) through teacher assessments and school records of the children's academic performance; and (c) from official records of standard achievement test scores maintained by the Board of Education of the City of New York.

Because the sample was large, physically mobile, and geographically dispersed, a major effort was made to keep track of the subjects, particularly after the children moved from the day care centers into public and private elementary schools. In addition, special procedures were devised to monitor the size and selectivity of attrition; during the fifth year of the study, social-emotional data were available on 74% of the boys and 79% of the girls, and standard achievement test scores were obtained for 66% of the boys and 73% of the girls, thus giving us a sizeable sample to work with even in the final year of the investigation. Although we detected a slight trend for the more disturbed children to drop out of the project and some indication that the girls who remained in the study were socially more disadvantaged than girls who were lost from the sample, there was little reason for concern that sample attrition introduced a bias that was likely to affect unduly the findings of the study.

Preliminary studies. The two patterns of disturbed behavior (recessive and acting-out) had been identified repeatedly during the last 50 years by innumerable researchers as the major types of emotional disorders in children. However, each team of investigators had generally applied their own terminology to the syndromes which emerged from their particular study. Therefore, before embarking on the five-year longitudinal investigation, for practical as well as theoretical reasons, we undertook a study to determine whether the different labels referred to the same or at least very similar dimensions of functioning. We found a high degree of congruence between corresponding factor dimensions from four instruments developed independently by three investigators. These results provided *empirical* evidence of the generality of the two-factor model of social-emotional functioning. It is rare in social science for a phenomenon to reappear with such regularity. We shall return to this point presently.

With the generality of the two-factor approach in clinical and mental health research thus underscored, we carried out a study to ascertain whether the two factor dimensions which had emerged from our instruments had clinical relevance. The data showed that the syndromes differentiated children with known psychiatric disorders from "normal" children; that, within the normal group, they discriminated among youngsters at varying levels of health and disturbance; and that they predicted to indices which in the past have been found to be valid clinical indicators, i.e., teachers' global ratings of children's functioning.

We proceeded to formulate hypotheses for the longitudinal study within the framework of previous research findings and our own clinical experience and judgment.

Data analyses for the longitudinal study. The large size of the longitudinal study sample enabled us to carry out a number of multivariate analyses to test the hypotheses. There were two classes of outcome criteria: emotional impairment measures and school achievement variables. The emotional impairment measures were (a) the dimensions of the two-factor model of social-emotional functioning (Interest-Participation versus Apathy-Withdrawal and Cooperation-Compliance versus Anger-Defiance), (b) a dimension of functioning pertinent to a classroom setting (High versus Low Task Orientation), assessed only in elementary school, and (c) two global ratings which indicated general level of functioning (Global Impairment) and need of therapeutic intervention (Referral). For the sake of convenience, the syndrome designations were shortened to Apathy-Withdrawal, Anger-Defiance, and Low Task Orientation, where feasible. Of course, when the focus was specifically on healthy functioning, the labels of the positive poles of the dimensions were used in reporting results.

The academic attainment variables consisted of (a) the scores on standardized tests (Metropolitan School Readiness Test [available only for the oldest group]; Verbal Achievement and Arithmetic Achievement, as measured by the Metropolitan Achievement Tests), (b) a teacher rating of school performance (Academic Standing), (c) a score to indicate whether the child

was in the appropriate grade for his age (Grade Placement), and
(d) a score to indicate whether the child was in a slow, average,
or fast class (Level Within Grade).

We selected as predictor variables five demographic factors,
five emotional impairment measures, and one variable related to
achievement. The demographic variables were age, sex, and three
variables relevant to disadvantaged status—social class, race-
ethnicity, and family intactness. The emotional impairment
variables were the same as those used as criterion measures. The
achievement variable (Verbal Fluency) was not an index of
academic attainment but was designed to yield a rough measure
of intelligence.

A major flaw in some studies is the failure to realize that a
specific outcome may not be caused by the effects of the
predictor under study but rather by a third factor which
influenced both the dependent and the independent variable.
For example, if the various syndrome variables measured the
same behavior rather than unique and different facets of
functioning, we would draw unwarranted conclusions regarding
persistence of specific types of emotional impairment or the
differential relationships between type of disorder and underachievement. Or, if home background and social-emotional
functioning were interrelated, a correlation between disturbance
at the first point in data collection and disturbance at a later age
might be misleading because the demographic variable might be
responsible for maintaining the same level of functioning over
the course of time. Or, if the three variables relevant to
disadvantaged status were interconnected, a linkage between,
e.g., race-ethnicity and underachievement might be a spurious
consequence produced by the relationship between race-ethnicity
and social class.

Accordingly, for the longitudinal predictions, our procedure
was to test *every independent variable for its partial relationship
to each dependent variable after all relevant others were
controlled for*. This was done for two time periods: In the case
of the investigation of longitudinal persistence of emotional
impairment, the two periods were from preschool through
fourth grade and from early to later elementary school; in the
case of the prediction of academic underachievement, the two

periods were from preschool to third grade and within-elementary school.

A shortage of funds affected the mode of data analysis by limiting the number of hierarchical multiple regression analyses that could be carried out; in some instances, we employed simple and partial correlational analyses and cross-tabulations.

As we presented our data and interpretations, we pointed out agreement or discrepancies between our results and those of other studies. Age trends and sex differences in social-emotional functioning and academic attainment were singled out for intensive analysis before we turned our attention to the effects of the disadvantaged status variables.

Sex and age differences in social-emotional functioning and academic attainment

In line with our expectations based on previous research, we found that at every age level boys were more disturbed than girls. Sex differences were largest on the global ratings and the two syndromes tapping acting-out behavior—Anger-Defiance and Low Task Orientation. On Apathy-Withdrawal, sex differences were smaller and diminished further with age.

We were surprised to observe a marked increase in pathology, particularly in boys, as the children grew older. The rising level of disturbance was evident on all five criterion measures for boys and on Apathy-Withdrawal and Referral for girls.

Both boys and girls also showed increasing disparity between actual and expected academic functioning during the first four years of elementary school.

The burden which the mounting emotional difficulties and educational failures of the children placed on the teachers were reflected in the exponential increase in the percentage of children with high Referral ratings between day care and fourth grade. The percentage of girls whom the teachers perceived to require intervention rose from 15% to over 35%; the percentage of boys, from 20% to close to 60%.

An increase in emotional disturbance when the children entered elementary school would not have been surprising. School makes new adaptive demands on children, and the stress may produce signs of disturbance (see Caplan, 1955; Lindeman, 1944). The persistent level of more impaired functioning, however, coupled with the decline in academic performance, is a matter of grave concern. Looking at the data in the framework of Biber and her colleagues' (see Minuchin et al., 1969) view of the role of the socio-educational milieu, one cannot escape the possible conclusion that the New York City public school system is detrimental to the mental health of its pupils. Of course, the negative impact of factors in the community, beyond the family and the school, cannot be ruled out as a possible explanation of the findings.

Epidemiology of emotional impairment and academic underachievement

We anticipated that the early environment of socially disadvantaged children would have a deleterious effect on their social-emotional functioning. By and large, the data did not support the assumption. Small but significant correlations indicated that broken family life predicted to high scores on Anger-Defiance and Low Task Orientation for boys and that low social-class level predicted to high Apathy-Withdrawal ratings for girls but there was little evidence connecting emotional impairment to minority-group membership. The correlations between broken home and boys' acting-out behavior and between lower-class background and girls' recessive behavior tended to increase gradually over time. The trend suggests that either social systems outside the family may impinge adversely on social-emotional functioning or the parents' disadvantaged status may interact with other determinants in the larger social milieu to produce psychopathology.

Since both a comprehensive review of the literature (see Dohrenwend & Dohrenwend, 1969) and the large-scale Manhattan Midtown Project (see Srole et al., 1962) have pointed to a strong inverse relationship between social status and prevalence of emotional disorders among adults, research is urgently needed to determine at what age level and under what circumstances the correlations become strong.

In comparison to the limited role of the disadvantaged status variables in children's social-emotional functioning, these background factors were found to play a larger part in their cognitive functioning: (a) Consistent with past research findings, we anticipated and found that as social class level declined, cognition deficit increased. (b) To our surprise, minority-group status was similarly linked to underachievement. We had supposed that after the effects of social class and family intactness had been statistically removed, the influence of the race and ethnic variables on school performance would become minimal. (c) Broken family life was related to deficiency in mathematics but not to verbal skills.

In short, the variables relevant to the advantaged-disadvantaged continuum did not show the same relationship to the achievement criteria as to the measures of social-emotional functioning.

Longitudinal persistence of emotional impairment

In accordance with our expectations, we found persistence of specific type of impairment, i.e., a child who was disturbed on one syndrome early in life was likely to exhibit the same pattern of pathology some years hence. The finding emerged from both the hierarchical regression and the simple correlational analyses. The partial syndrome-to-syndrome correlations were of modest-to-moderate magnitude in both prediction periods. When correlations were examined at successive age levels, stability of functioning was found to increase with age.

The simple cross-syndrome correlations declined over time: Correlations between Apathy-Withdrawal and the two syndromes became very small, and those between Anger-Defiance and Low Task Orientation were only moderate in size. However, in the hierarchical multiple regression analyses, a number of the cross-syndrome correlations, though small, were statistically significant although consistently lower than the same-syndrome correlations. The significant r_p's indicated that Cooperation-Compliance predicted to Apathy-Withdrawal across both time periods; Interest-Participation predicted to Anger-Defiance and Low Task Orientation predicted to Apathy-Withdrawal in the within-elementary school analysis. We will account for these cross-syndrome correlations in terms of the circumplex model of child behavior.

It will be recalled that Interest-Participation versus Apathy-Withdrawal and Cooperation-Compliance versus Anger-Defiance accounted for the major sources of the variation on the Symptom Checklist and the Social Competence Scale (see chapter 3). The factor score for each of the two factors was composed of many items. Previous work by Emmerich (1977) and Schaefer (1961, 1971), among others, has disclosed that when these items are plotted in such a way as to show the extent to which every item has a loading on each of the two factors, the items arrange themselves to form a circle, or a circumplex. A hypothetical situation is presented in Figure 9.

According to Emmerich, social-emotional development can take the form of both consistent behavior and change over time. This approach encompasses two kinds of correlation coefficients: (a) a stability coefficient—namely, the correlation between the same syndrome measured at one age and again some years later, and (b) a transformation coefficient—namely, the correlation between one syndrome measured at one age and a different syndrome measured some time later. A high stability coefficient indicates consistency in functioning, and a high transformation coefficient represents behavioral change. When a low (or in our case, moderate) stability correlation occurs in conjunction with a significant transformation coefficient, the child's behavior is changing "qualitatively in a way that links an earlier disposition to a later one" (p. 21).

Emmerich postulated that "behavioral changes on a particular gradient will be sequentially ordered in accordance with the proximity principle" (p. 21). If we consider the circumplex such a gradient, a child identified initially as high on Cooperation-Compliance would change in the direction either of Interest-Participation or Apathy-Withdrawal, and a child who showed early signs of Interest-Participation would move in the direction of either Cooperation-Compliance or Anger-Defiance.

Our data showed that changes were in a maladaptive direction, with the cooperative-compliant child becoming shy and withdrawn and the socially outgoing child becoming aggressive and hostile. We hypothesize that the quality of the environment determines the direction of change along the circumplex gradient. We have previously inferred that the

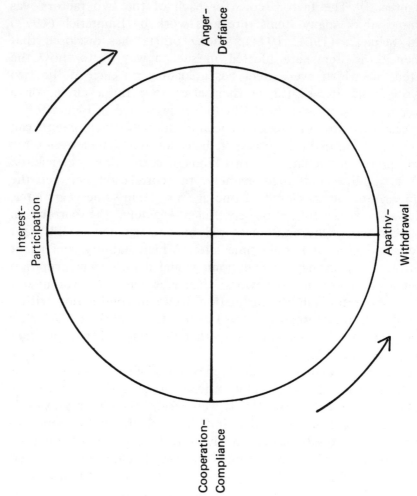

FIG. 9. A hypothetical model of social-emotional functioning.

increase in pathology in our sample over time (see chapter 6) was probable evidence that the schools of New York provided an unfavorable climate for the children's emotional development. The shift from Cooperation-Compliance to Apathy-Withdrawal and from Interest-Participation to Anger-Defiance can be interpreted as evidence in support of this view since both changes were from healthy to disturbed behavior. A shift from Anger-Defiance to Interest-Participation or from Apathy-Withdrawal to Cooperation-Compliance (i.e., in the direction of health) was not possible because the same two axes are involved. Future research is of course needed to corroborate the selective move from healthy to disturbed patterns of functioning in maladaptive settings or from disturbed to healthy behavior in a constructive environment.

It is possible to add a third independent axis, e.g., High versus Low Task Orientation, to the circumplex model. This implies a spherical scheme since the Task Orientation dimension and Interest-Participation versus Apathy-Withdrawal are orthogonal to each other. Without going into the complexities of the spherical model, if we bear in mind Emmerich's proposition that behavioral change occurs in sequential order according to the proximity principle, the shift from early Low Task Orientation to later Apathy-Withdrawal becomes plausible. This change was from one disturbed pattern to another.

Children at risk. The demographic variables and the emotional impairment measures jointly accounted for 25% to 35% of the variance of the three syndromes in the preschool through fourth grade data analysis (percentages varied with the syndrome) and 26% to 41% of the variance of the three syndrome measures in the early to later elementary school data analysis. These percentages are sufficiently high to identify groups of children who are likely to show pathology of a particular type. To the best of our knowledge, this is the first study in which prediction to specific syndromes of disturbance has been accomplished.

In addition to analyzing longitudinal persistence through simple, partial, and multiple correlations, we used cross-tabulations to obtain collateral evidence that early identification of children at risk was feasible. We divided the youngsters into groups of varying levels of disturbance and health: Those whose scores fell into the top 25% of the distribution were designated the most disturbed group on each syndrome, and those whose scores were in the bottom 25% of the distribution were considered the healthiest group on each syndrome. Cross-tabulations of the data from each age level to every other showed that the median rate of persistence of disturbance for all time periods covered in the analysis was 45% for each of the three syndrome measures; conversely, the median rate of remission was 55%. For healthy functioning, persistence ranged between 38% and 49% (depending on the syndrome), and consequently, change in level of functioning (i.e., deterioration) varied from 51% to 62%. In general, stability of behavior decreased and remission increased as the time lapse between rating occasions became longer.

The 25% cut-off point used in the present study was an arbitrary number in which we have no vested interest. The concepts of "selectivity" and "predictive range" which Stott (1960) developed for his work on the identification of delinquents are of relevance here. "Selectivity" refers to the proportion of all cases who have been accurately identified as positives, and "predictive range" refers to the proportion of all true positives in the sample who have been spotted. As Stott pointed out, "The higher the [degree of] selectivity, the smaller the range, and conversely. In other words, a high score criterion will pick out few among the total number of delinquents, but nearly all will be correctly picked; on the other hand, a low score criterion will embrace a good percent of the delinquents' total but include a large number of non-delinquents" (p. 195).

We assume that if we had used a higher cut-off score for the disturbed and a lower cut-off score for the healthy children, the rate of persistence would have been higher and the rate of remission, lower. The optimal cut-off point depends on the purpose which the screening process is to serve. If an intervention program is to be directed at *all* emotionally impaired children, there should be no cut-off point at all. If, for the sake of efficiency, the intervention effort is to be limited to youngsters who are at highest risk, a high score criterion should be set; most of the target population will be reached although some may escape the net.

Persistence of recessive as compared to acting-out behavior. Both the longitudinal correlations and the cross-tabulations dealing with children at risk showed that acting-out behavior, as measured by Anger-Defiance and Low Task Orientation, was consistently more stable than recessive behavior, as measured by Apathy-Withdrawal. We have previously obtained the same finding in a study in which we assessed both cross-situational and longitudinal persistence of the two behavior patterns (Kohn & Rosman, 1973b). In a more recent study in which we focused on cross-situational stability (Koretzky, 1976; Koretzky & Kohn, 1976), the recessive behavior (Factor I) correlations were also less robust than the acting-out behavior (Factor II) correlations. (These data appear in Table 10.1 later in the present chapter.)

The cross-tabulations dealing with children at risk gave us the opportunity to determine the extent to which the healthy or disturbed pole of each dimension contributed to stability of functioning or lack thereof. As stated earlier, the disturbed ends of all three dimensions showed approximately the same rate of persistence over time. On the other hand, Interest-Participation (the polar opposite of Apathy-Withdrawal) was less stable than the healthy poles of the other two dimensions. Therefore, it is reasonable to conclude that the lower longitudinal persistence of Factor I is primarily attributable to the lower stability of Interest-Participation. The findings imply that, as the most delicate of the syndromes, Interest-Participation requires the most careful environmental nurturance if it is to be maintained and strengthened.

Relationship between emotional impairment and academic underachievement

The data supported our assumptions that psychopathology existing prior to entrance into elementary school would predict to academic difficulties and that specific syndromes would be differentially related to underachievement.

When preschool was the point of prediction, Apathy-Withdrawal was strongly associated with poor cognitive functioning on Verbal Achievement, Arithmetic Achievement, Academic Standing, Grade Placement, and Level Within Grade. Anger-Defiance was less strongly related to the achievement criteria: The syndrome predicted to poor performance on the arithmetic tests and, to a lesser extent, to low scores on the verbal tests but not to the other outcome measures.

When first grade was the point of prediction, Apathy-Withdrawal and Low Task Orientation (not assessed in preschool) were implicated in educational failure on every criterion variable. Cooperation-Compliance (the polar opposite of Anger-Defiance) was related to difficulties with math and to low Academic Standing ratings.

We hypothesize that impairment on Apathy-Withdrawal and Low Task Orientation leads to underachievement in the following ways: Learning is a function of, among other things, exposure to environmental stimuli and the child's ability to process information and formulate assumptions about the world in which he lives, i.e., thought processes. The shy and inhibited child isolates himself from contact with people, events, and objects, and he is listless and sluggish in his mode of thinking. The hyperactive and restless child's interactions with his surroundings are too brief and superficial for him to acquire knowledge and develop intellectual skills; he has a short attention span, cannot concentrate, and his mental processes are disorganized.

An analysis of the curvilinear relationship between the two syndromes and performance on the standardized achievement tests showed that the whole spectrum of social-emotional functioning from health to disturbance was involved in classroom learning: Not only were emotionally impaired children handicapped in school achievement but emotionally healthy children enjoyed an advantage in mastering academic subjects. If we relate the positive ends of the dimensions to academic attainment along the lines hypothesized above, the child who is inquisitive about the world around him interacts frequently with people and objects and has an active mind. The task-involved child has systematic contacts with his environment and thinks in an organized way.

The Cooperation-Compliance versus Anger-Defiance linkage with underachievement is somewhat ambiguous, and correlations were not as robust as those between the other syndromes and underachievement. It is possible that the cooperative-compliant child is so obedient and "good" that he has given up initiative.

Also, the fact that Cooperation-Compliance predicted to Apathy-Withdrawal, which in turn is related to under-achievement, may have some bearing on the issue.

Studies involving young children (see Emmerich, 1977; Richards & McCandless, 1972) have found Apathy-Withdrawal to be associated with cognitive deficits; on the other hand, investigations with preadolescents and adolescent samples (see President's Commission on Law Enforcement and Administration of Justice, 1967; Rutter et al., 1970) have yielded evidence that Anger-Defiance was related to school failure. Research is urgently needed to shed further light on the relationship between type of emotional impairment and underachievement; specifically, (a) whether the relationship changes with age, or (b) whether the findings on the older subjects were primarily due to special or deviant study samples.

The demographic variables, emotional impairment measures, and Verbal Fluency jointly accounted for about 25% of the variance of the standard achievement test scores from preschool to third grade and for nearly 30% of the variance of these measures in the within-elementary school period. The percentages are large enough to identify groups of children who are at risk of underachievement.

Usefulness of the two-factor model as a research tool

On the whole, the present study reached its objective of demonstrating the practical value of the two-factor model of social-emotional functioning in clinical and mental health research.

We showed that each dimension was a valid clinical indicator, was relatively independent of the other, predicted uniquely to itself, and was differentially related to underachievement. The syndromes were found to cover almost the entire range of behavior generally included under the rubric of emotional impairment in a classroom setting (as indicated by the fact that in the hierarchical multiple regression analyses, Global Impairment and Referral accounted for very small amounts of the variance after the syndromes had been partialed out). In that respect our results were very similar to those of Rutter et al. (1970) who found that neurotic disorders (Apathy-Withdrawal), antisocial disorders (Anger-Defiance), and cases showing both neurotic and antisocial symptoms accounted for 90% of all the disturbed children whom they examined in their Isle of Wight study. Since the dimensions were bipolar, the entire range of functioning—from healthy to disturbed—was measured.

Naturally, it would be naive to assume that the complexity of children's behavior can be encompassed within a two- or even three-dimensional framework. Yet it is challenging to test this parsimonious model to its very limits (validity, reliability, longitudinal stability, differential predictive value, antecedent relationships, amont of variance of behavior accounted for, cross-setting generality, etc.) and to determine how potent it is. Judging by the findings of the present study as well as others reported in the literature, the model is potent.

Moreover, it is possible to stay within the two-dimensional schema and yet go beyond it. How is this possible? The reader will recall our earlier discussion of the circumplex model; we showed how additional personality concepts can be incorporated into the model at different angles and identified at various points along the hypothetical ring around two axes. In that way, the researcher has an economical and psychologically meaningful way of describing personality functioning, and yet he can make it as complex as he desires.

Cross-Situational Generality of Social-Emotional Functioning

In many previous investigations (e.g., Ackerson, Hewitt & Jenkins, Robins) the diagnosis of emotional disturbance was based on behavior and symptoms which the child manifested in different settings (home, school, community). The information was obtained from different people (parents, teachers, guidance counselors, social workers) by means of different methods (interviews, ratings, testing procedures, school reports). While the use of multiple data sources provided a broad index of the child's functioning, the very diversity of the data sources and the lack of standardization from case to case raise questions of validity and reliability from the researcher's point of view. Moreover—and this is the issue at stake here—the data-gathering procedure obscured the fact that a child may behave in one way in one setting, such as the home, and act quite differently in another environment, such as the school.

The desire for data that were (a) more systematic, and (b) on normal rather than disturbed children led investigators (Peterson, Schaefer) to focus on the school as a research setting. This was the approach we followed in our own work.

The question arises to what extent it is possible to generalize from classroom functioning to behavior in another setting. Peterson (1968) became discouraged some years ago when he found modest correlations between the child's behavior in school, as rated by his teacher, and his behavior at home, as rated by his parents (see Peterson, Becker, Shoemaker, Luria, & Hellmer, 1961). We have previously criticized Peterson's approach (Kohn & Rosman, 1973b) by pointing out that the modest correlations may have been due in part to the procedures employed: Teachers and parents rated the children on exactly the same behavior items in the two settings yet the items did not necessarily have the same meaning in the two environments. Substantial cross-situational correlations require that test items be appropriate not only to the trait being sampled but also to the setting in which the trait is assessed.

Peterson's (1968) conclusion that the two-factor model did not meet the test of cross-setting generality was in line with the *Zeitgeist*—the environment rather than the individual was viewed as the determinant of the individual's behavior. This position was consistent with the situationism of the psychological ecologists (see Barker & Wright, 1955) and with the operant conditioning and behavior modification approaches (see, e.g., Risley & Baer, 1973). Mischel (1968) was able to marshal a considerable amount of evidence that generality of traits across situations was minimal.

In contrast, we found evidence in two recent studies that the two-factor model had cross-setting generality. We obtained correlations of moderate size between behavior in the classroom and in a test-taking situation (Kohn & Rosman, 1973b) and correlations of considerable magnitude between conduct in

Table 10.1 Stability of Factor Dimensions across Settings

School ratings	Residence ratings	
	Factor I	Factor II
Factor I	.40**	−.08
Factor II	−.27*	.60**

Note.−*N* = 110.

Factor I = Interest-Participation versus Apathy-Withdrawal; Factor II = Cooperation-Compliance versus Anger-Defiance.

  *$p \leqslant .01$.
  **$p \leqslant .001$.

school and in residence at an institution for delinquent children (Koretzky, 1976; Koretzky & Kohn, 1976). The latter results are shown in Table 10.1.

A major reason for these encouraging results is the fact that the dimensions of the two-factor model account for substantial portions of the variance of social-emotional functioning. Broad, higher-order factors are more replicable than narrow factors (Peterson, 1960, 1965). Researchers working with narrow factors should not be surprised if they obtain low cross-situational correlation coefficients. Another reason is that the measuring instruments were carefully worded to fit the setting in which behavior was assessed.

Yet at best the correlations account for 36% of the variance. Why not more? because behavior may vary from setting to setting. An extreme example was the discovery of Ricks and Berry (1970) that some preschizophrenic boys acted withdrawn in school and rebellious at home (see chapter 2). However, cross-situational variability may be a reflection of the child's tendency to respond to changes in environmental contingencies and not only an indication of unpredictability or absence of enduring personality attributes (see Bem & Allen, 1974).

Social-Emotional Functioning and the Environment

We will now elaborate on the point made earlier in the chapter regarding the "enormous" generality of the two factors of social-emotional functioning in studies on children and adolescents.

In a previous paper (Kohn, 1975) we hypothesized that the two dimensions of social-emotional functioning were related to two major situational determinants. Stern (1970) analyzed learning environments using Murray's (1938) need-press model as the conceptual foundation for his work. In this model "need" is a characteristic of the individual and refers to his drives, wishes, motives, etc.; "press" is a characteristic of the external situation and refers to resources, opportunities, expectations of others, etc. Stern differentiated between two kinds of press—"anabolic," represented by stimuli which facilitate growth and self-enhancement (e.g., intellectual climate) and "catabolic," represented by stimuli which place constraints on personal development and effectiveness (e.g., organizational structure).

We agree with the general concept of Stern's anabolic dimension but to say that controls are necessarily antithetical to personal development and effectiveness is to prejudge the issue. A different, and perhaps more helpful, formulation is that a social system, to be viable, must have two fundamental characteristics:

1. The system must provide opportunities for personal satisfactions and furnish environmental supports and means to put these satisfactions within the reach of its members.
2. The system must provide norms, rules, and procedures to guide the social interactions of its members and ensure the orderly functioning of the system. Without organizational stability, the individual is too preoccupied with self-preservation to seek self-fulfillment.

These two components were found by Roff (1949) who did a factor analysis of parent behavior toward young children, as measured by the Fels Behavior Rating Scale (although the scales subsumed under the second factor dealt not so much with the prescription of rules as with the way in which they were enforced). The negative side of these dimensions may be seen in Hewitt and Jenkins' (1946) family situational patterns, described in chapter 2: Family repression allows few opportunities for personal satisfaction while parental rejection and parental negligence are characterized by absence of system-maintaining home processes.

Of particular interest is the investigation by Prescott and Jones (1967) who studied the social climate of day care centers and identified by factor analysis two major patterns of teacher behavior. Pattern I was labeled "Encouragement/Restriction;" it was the strongest pattern and was bipolar. The factor described the alternative ways in which teachers reacted to the feelings and behavior of the children. "Those teachers who accept and elaborate on children's behavior account for high positive loadings on encouragement and on lessons in consideration and creativity" (p. 117). The negative pole denoted "restriction and use of control and restraint, behaviors which characterize teachers who respond repressively to children's feelings and behavior" (p. 118).

The similarity of the positive pole to our hypothesized situational component #1 and of the negative pole to Hewitt and Jenkins' family repression environment is clear.

Prescott and Jones' Pattern II was called "Conformity to Routine" and reflected the extent to which the teacher was concerned with enabling the children to adapt to the routines of social living. Guidance, structuring, and teacher direction loaded high on this factor. Conformity to Routine corresponds to our hypothesized situational component #2. The dimension was unipolar, very likely due to inadequate sampling of behaviors suggesting rejection or neglect.

In addition to the variables measuring teacher behavior, Prescott and Jones collected information on many other variables, one of which is particularly pertinent to this discussion. The investigators called this variable, "Children's Responses;" actually, the 5-point scale could be described more aptly as measuring the children's level of interest and involvement since a high score denoted genuine interest and exceptional involvement in the activities of the classroom, and a low score was indicative of disinterest, boredom, restlessness, and lethargy. In a rough global way, the variable is analogous to the Interest-Participation versus Apathy-Withdrawal dimension of the present study.

This index was found to be highly correlated ($r = .70$) with Teacher Pattern I, Encouragement/Restriction, lending support to the hypothesis that environmental factors, in this case the social climate of a classroom and the teacher's style of presenting the curriculum, are important determinants of children's social-emotional functioning.

The variable was found to be less strongly related ($r = -.29$) to Teacher Pattern II, Conformity to Routine, indicating that the environmental dimensions have differential impact on children's functioning. These results suggest that strong emphasis on living within rules and limits has a mildly inhibiting effect on the interest-disinterest dimension whereas children's attentiveness and participation can be fostered in a climate which optimizes opportunities for growth and ego-actualization.

It is unfortunate that Prescott and Jones did not have a global rating tapping the Cooperation-Compliance versus Anger-Defiance dimension. We hypothesize that this index would have been strongly correlated with Conformity to Routine and shown only a modest association with Encouragement/Restriction.

To sum up, we believe that two basic dimensions of the environment set the stage for two major adaptive demands that every social setting makes of its members: how to utilize the opportunities for personal development and how to live within the norms and regulations that maintain an orderly group process. The way in which the child "chooses" to cope with these demands determines his level of Interest-Participation versus Apathy-Withdrawal and his level of Cooperation-Compliance versus Anger-Defiance. We hypothesize that it is the wide generality of the two adaptive demands that accounts for the wide generality of the two-factor model of social-emotional functioning.

And when the child exercises the same options in different environments, we find cross-situational generality.

The Two-Factor Model and Risk Research

In recent years there has been an escalation of interest in risk research. To the researcher, one of the important issues has been the methods that different investigators have employed for seeking out antecedents of emotional impairment and systematically following developmental processes.

It may be worthwhile to review briefly four research strategies and weigh the advantages and disadvantages of each before turning the spotlight on the present study to point out the implications of our methodology for risk research.

Research strategies

"Follow-back" method. "Follow-back" is a retrospective approach in which the starting point is the disordered adult, and the researcher examines the person's past to uncover events and symptoms which may anticipate later psychopathology or academic difficulties. The retrospective review may be based on data derived from interviews with patients, peers, and parents or, preferably, on records maintained by more "neutral" observers, e.g., school data, teachers' assessments, and court, child guidance clinic, or hospital case records. This approach was adopted by Watt et al. (1970), as reported in chapter 2.

The principal advantages of the follow-back method are that all cases are salient because the initial selection is based on the specific status of deviance the researcher wishes to investigate, and the methodology allows for flexibility in generating and testing hypotheses as new leads appear. But the disadvantages are numerous:

1. Samples are biased, especially if the subjects are drawn from child guidance clinic sources (i.e., in this population there is a disproportionate ratio of boys to girls and of angry-defiant to apathetic-withdrawn children as well as a disproportionate number of youngsters with learning disabilities).

2. If data on childhood events are gathered from patients and family respondents, the information usually lacks validity because of memory lapses or memory coloration. "People tend to remember and report items that help make sense of the outcome or excuse it" (Robins, 1966, p. 7).

3. Relevant data, such as clinic, school, court, or police records, may not be available or, if available, these data are

often inadequate, lacking important factual information and/or containing content that is biased, highly impressionistic, or imprecise.

4. Often control groups are not readily available. When they are, the data on control subjects may suffer from the same shortcomings as those on study subjects or may be even more deficient since these children may not have come to the attention of clinics or courts although they would have school records. Moreover, a control group chosen on the basis of adult outcome will show differences on many childhood variables from the study sample, and it is difficult to tell which particular childhood variables contributed to adverse adult outcome.

5. The approach focuses only on cases at risk who turned out to be deviant; others who were equally at risk and showed remission are lost track of.

6. The investigator must be cautious about drawing conclusions regarding the antecedent-consequent relationship, as will be illustrated presently.

Consequently, the ability to generalize findings that emerge from follow-back studies is severely limited.

"Follow-up" method. "Follow-up" is a prospective strategy in which the starting point is the disturbed child, and the researcher studies the adult to assess his present status. The reader will recall that several long-term follow-up studies of children who were impaired on one or both major syndrome patterns were described in chapter 2. The number of such investigations has been limited because:

1. A very sizeable initial sample is needed so as to identify in later years a sufficiently large number of criterion cases to enable the researcher to test specific hypotheses and make generalizations.

2. Whatever the nature of the institutional population that is selected for study, the drawbacks noted previously with respect to sample bias, questionable quality of input data, and inability to generalize the findings pertain.

3. Since many years have elapsed since the time the child came to the attention of the clinic or institution and the time when outcome data are available, the researcher will

encounter difficulties in locating subjects, especially in a mobile society.

Nevertheless, the follow-up approach is superior to the follow-back approach. A telling illustration of the point is provided by Sameroff and Chandler (1975) who made a very thorough and comprehensive review of the literature dealing with risk factors operative during the prenatal and early postnatal periods. They stated, "Retrospective investigations showed that individuals suffering a wide range of disorders, from cerebral palsy to mental retardation and schizophrenia, were more likely to have experienced complicated births than individuals without the disorders" (p. 232) and gave the impression "of having established clear relationships between pregnancy and delivery complications and later deviance" (p. 236). "The general findings of prospective studies have not, however, supported the inference drawn from these retrospective studies that such birth complications provide direct, causal explanations for later disorders" (p. 232). A majority of babies who experienced perinatal problems and who were followed from infancy through school age proved to have "normal developmental outcomes" (p. 236). Sameroff and Chandler concluded that whether difficulties around birth led to later problems depended on the caretaking environment in which the children were reared. "As a general rule, only when information regarding the nature of the subsequent caretaking environment has also been taken into account have such long-range predictions about the later consequences of pregnancy and birth complications been successful" (p. 218).

"Longitudinal" method. Another type of prospective study has traditionally been called the "longitudinal" approach (labeled "follow-through" research by Garmezy, 1974) in which the investigator collects data on study (and control) subjects in childhood and follows the youngsters over a period of time until he is ready to measure the particular outcomes in which he is interested. The longitudinal investigation may be of short- or long-term duration.

This method is ideal for studying child development and specifically, the etiology of disturbed as well as healthy functioning. The researcher can start out with an unbiased sample of the population, and, with the increasing sophistication in the field, he is likely to know which variables are cogent and can be selective. The investigator can fix the time intervals between measurements and observe continuities or discontinuities in behavior at successive age levels as well as over a stretch of years. The question of stability of behavior over time is a particularly important issue in risk research. Furthermore, the method permits the investigator to draw conclusions about causal directions although he must always entertain alternative hypotheses which may vitiate his conclusions because he is not introducing variables experimentally but is observing time sequences.

The chief drawbacks of the method are:

1. A large sample must be followed since a longitudinal study is bound to generate a large number of cases who will not be index cases. For example, in the present study children who were initially very disturbed showed remission, and some children who were initially very healthy became disturbed. Actually, such cases need not be a nuisance to the investigator but rather, as was pointed out in chapter 8, youngsters showing change in level of functioning are in themselves worthwhile focal points for future research.

2. There is the problem whether the measures selected at the beginning of the study will appear adequate at the conclusion of the study; sometimes investigators lack, to quote Escalona and Leitsch (1952), "the very facts which they would currently find of greatest interest but which played no significant part in their thinking when the longitudinal study was begun" (p. 25). Moreover, the relative inflexibility of the methodology makes it difficult to test new hypotheses since the researcher is limited to the data which have been collected.

3. Such studies involve large expenditures and require a long-term commitment on the part of the investigator.

"Convergence approach". A fourth technique for conducting risk research is what Bell (1953) termed the "convergence approach" which consists of integrating the longitudinal method

with a series of successive cross-sectional studies. Before elaborating on this method, the cross-sectional procedure requires a brief examination.

A series of successive cross-sectional studies entails the simultaneous gathering of data on different children at different ages and evaluating developmental trends. The findings may suggest new hypotheses which can be tested in further studies so that the process of studying antecedent-consequent behavior is speeded up. However, the possibility remains that observed changes in age groups are a function of differences other than age between the groups studied. Moreover, interactions of which the researcher may be unaware may influence the outcome (see Wenar & Wenar, 1963, p. 702).

Under the convergence approach, the researcher tests different age groups recurrently over short periods of time so that the data of each age cohort bridge into the data of the next age cohort. He thus obtains information on the dependent variable (behavior) for short-term intervals as well as data which "will permit an answer to the question of whether the shorter curves for each age span may reasonably be combined into a curve covering the entire age period" (Bell, 1953, p. 147). If so, the investigator can estimate persistence of behavior over several years in a much briefer span of time.

Wynne (1972) is currently applying the convergence method to risk studies. A five-year study will compare groups at risk (as defined by mother's psychiatric status) and control children at ages 4, 7, and 10 years. In the fourth year of the study, those who were initially in the 4- and 7-year-old groups will be 7 and 10 years old, respectively. They can thus serve on retesting as cross-validating samples of the two older original subgroups. As Garmezy (1974) noted, "Within the span of 4 years an estimate may be possible of the developmental characteristics of the variables under study for a period extending from ages 4 to 13" (p. 57).

Bell conceded that the convergence approach is not always appropriate, however. The researcher who is interested in the cumulative impact of an independent variable (e.g., long-term effects of annual guidance and counseling services for school children) must use the longitudinal method.

Contributions of the present study

The longitudinal project reported in this book exemplifies a promising new approach to risk research. We started with a very large sample ($N = 1,232$) that was randomly selected from the population of children. We approached but did not quite reach the ideal of a completely unbiased sample since youngsters in public-funded day care centers are not truly representative of the entire population of children, i.e., upper-class families and intact families are underrepresented.

Our subjects were neither clinic patients nor, as in prospective studies of children at risk of schizophrenia cited by Garmezy, the offspring of psychiatrically ill parents. Rather, the children were "normal," i.e., there was a distribution ranging from healthy to disturbed. Consequently, the present approach was more likely to show the pattern of weaving in and out of disturbance than use of a risk sample based on emotional disturbance of parents would have done, and we were, therefore, in a position to generalize our findings to the population at large rather than to children already predisposed to risk.

One of the advantages of a large sample is that there are built-in control groups. Had additional funds been available, we could have made comparisons on a variety of indices (constitutional/genetic, familial, social) among the most disturbed, the healthiest, and the "average" subgroups (see chapter 8). Or we could have made these comparisons between youngsters whose emotional problems increased and youngsters whose social-emotional functioning improved over time.

We took yearly measurements and thus had a short-term as well as a longer-term perspective on stability of behavior at the conclusion of the study. While a major effort was required to keep track of the sample, data collection procedures were relatively simple and straightforward.

But the key point is that our central focus was on the two major dimensions which have proven themselves highly salient with respect to risk. Previous follow-up and follow-back studies dealt with deviant samples and, therefore, were highly limited in the generality of their findings. Early longitudinal studies of normal children (e.g., Macfarlane et al., 1954; Sanford, Adkins,

Miller, & Cobb, 1943) were largely exploratory in nature, wide in scope, and comprehensive in data collection because the investigators were (a) interested in the "whole child" (Sanford et al., 1943, p. 2), and (b) not sure which variables were likely to appear at later age levels. "We resolved to take into account as many factors as possible. Physiological, intellectual, personality and environmental aspects were roughly marked off for convenience. Within each of these fields numerous variables—the more significant ones, as it seemed—were selected, or when necessary defined, and observed by appropriate techniques" (Sanford et al., 1943, p. 3).

We showed that the two fundamental syndrome patterns, which are valid clinical entities, permit the identification of segments of the sample whose propensity for deficits in social-emotional and/or cognitive functioning makes them a target group most in need of intervention and most useful as subjects in etiological investigations.

Prospective View

Similar to the periodic reinvention of the wheel, behavioral scientists have rediscovered the two fundamental dimensions of functioning again and again and again. With the present study we have broadened the scope and applicability of the two-factor model. We have demonstrated the successful use of the longitudinal method to observe continuities and discontinuities in the behavior of children between the ages of 3 and 10 and to detect groups of children at risk of emotional impairment and/or academic underachievement. We have further demonstrated the utility of readily available sources of childhood information— namely, the teacher's knowledge of the children and also school records—in longitudinal research involving a very large sample.

The groundwork has now been laid for future studies in which the two-factor model can be the central focus of research into risk of disturbance and development of healthy behavior. A systematic research approach needs to address itself to the following issues:

Multi-setting assessments

One line of investigation should extend the two-factor model to social systems other than the classroom, particularly the family and the neighborhood peer group. With some exceptions, we do not yet have the methodology for the systematic assessment of Factor I and II functioning in other settings. As pointed out earlier in the chapter, it is not satisfactory to use the same scale items to rate a child's behavior in different situations; traits (e.g., interest or compliance) often express themselves in varied ways at home, among peers, or in the classroom.

To study cross-situational generality, therefore, systematic research instruments similar to those which have been developed for the rating of children's functioning in the classroom need to be developed for assessment of behavior with family members in the home and with peers in the neighborhood.

A global measure of Factor I and Factor II functioning should be derived either by pooling the respective Factor I and II scores from the different settings or by using the score from different environments as separate independent variables in a multiple regression approach in order to predict to a given criterion measure. It is plausible to assume that Factor I and II functioning based on behavior in a number of situations will be more stable and will lead to stronger predictions than ratings based on behavior in one setting only. The pooling of matched factor scores across settings (classroom and test-taking situation) enhanced longitudinal stability coefficients in a previous study by the author (Kohn & Rosman, 1973b; see chapter 8).

Data collected by different observers in a variety of environments over a span of four years also gave Kagan and Moss (1962) high longitudinal correlations (in the 60's and 70's) on four personality variables similar to our bipolar dimensions ("Social spontaneity" and "Withdrawal"; "Conformity" and "Aggression"). However, this evidence is not unambiguous since the stability coefficients may have been inflated by the fact that a single judge rated all observer data on these dimensions.

Our comments so far have rested on the assumption of congruence between factor scores across settings, i.e., that the child who is rated high on Apathy-Withdrawal in the classroom is likely to be rated high on Apathy-Withdrawal in the home. However, since, as noted earlier, stability coefficients have at best been found to account for 36% of the variance (see

Koretzky, 1976; Koretzky & Kohn, 1976), it is clear that there is also inconsistency in functioning across settings. The topic of consistency versus inconsistency in functioning in different environments is of major research interest. We should further explore such questions as: What factors in the child's make-up or in the social situation lead to stable or inconsistent behavior across settings? To what extent is stable or inconsistent behavior across settings related to later psychopathology? The latter question is more than an academic issue but has prognostic significance in the light of Ricks and Berry's findings that boys who manifested Anger-Defiance within the family and Apathy-Withdrawal within the community were at particularly high risk of becoming chronic schizophrenics as adults.

Garmezy has raised the point that it is important to examine what he called the *"locus of action* of behavior" (p. 52). This issue also is of more than theoretical interest because of its predictive value (Ricks and Berry reported that boys who showed violence and defiance against family members had a worse prognosis than boys who were aggressive and hostile toward peers).

The number of possible combinations of behavior assessed on two bipolar dimensions in even only two environments is enormous considering that the child may be consistent or inconsistent on Factor I across settings, consistent or inconsistent on Factor II across settings, and that the two factors are relatively independent of each other. This formulation suggests how little we know of the whole panorama of possible behavioral phenomena conceptualized along these lines.

Family variables related to risk

A second extension of the research pursued in the present study should be a risk-oriented analysis of the child's functioning in the family and the family network of which the child is a part. For example, Ricks and Berry found that not only was the presence of one or both symptom syndromes predictive of later schizophrenia but the nature of the parent-child relationship was an important determinant of the severity of subsequent pathology.

The two major family patterns of preschizophrenics were (a) "symbiotic union," which united parent and child "in a small island apart from the world" (p. 37) and tended to produce chronicity of impairment, and (b) "family sacrifice" or rejection, which was the dominant feature of the home atmosphere in which many of the released schizophrenics grew up. We assume it is not coincidental that disturbed functioning and a deviant family role existed simultaneously; rather the pathological family constellation maintained the disturbed behavior which eventually led to the schizophrenic break.

This raises the more general question of the ways in which the parent-child relationship and the family environment in which the child is embedded are implicated in the youngster's social-emotional development, for better or for worse. Bearing in mind the two situational determinants postulated earlier, we would expect emotional health to prevail if the familial system provides encouragement and support for the child's initiatives and gratification of his needs plus standards for the child's conduct and discipline to secure his compliance. Conversely, we hypothesize that early emotional difficulties will arise and persist when combined with and fostered by chronically adverse environmental circumstances of a psychological nature (as postulated by the model). Naturally, in future studies other potential determinants, such as genetic factors, demonstrable brain damage, and early symptoms of psychotic functioning, which maintain disturbed behavior should also be included in the research design.

Of equal research interest are the psychodynamic factors which produce shifts in functioning, either remission of symptoms or onset of pathology. Thus, we should further explore such questions as: Is the home life of children who recover more supportive and growth-promoting than that of children who remain disturbed? Are the families more responsive to the developmental tasks that the child has to solve during that particular period in his life? Conversely, under what conditions does a healthy youngster develop emotional problems?

Great advances in therapy might be possible if we knew what family events were related to remission from disturbance. We might then attempt to mobilize experimentally those family variables which are likely to have a favorable influence on outcome.

Research is needed not only on parental effects on the child's development but also on the contribution that the child makes to the familial interaction pattern. As has been repeatedly emphasized (see reviews of the literature by Bell, 1968, and Sameroff & Chandler, 1975; also, Wenar & Wenar, 1963; among others), the child is not necessarily a passive recipient of external forces but has stimulus value in evoking environmental responses.[29] The behavior of the child may predispose parents to warmth or hostility, to overprotectiveness or neglect. Sameroff and Chandler pointed out that children with "poor reproductive histories" tended to elicit poor caretaking responses from their parents, and it was this transaction between child and parents which placed the youngster at risk and contributed to developmental disorders. In other words, the characteristics of both parents and offspring must be considered in predicting a child's developmental outcome.

Emotional health

The present study focused on a phenomenon which has been largely neglected by researchers—namely, healthy functioning. We have shown that some children remained remarkably stable on the three dimensions over three- to five-year periods and thrived despite unfavorable social circumstances. Yet we know relatively little of the antecedents of emotional health.

One of the few investigators who has examined this issue is Baumrind (Baumrind, 1967; Baumrind & Black, 1967) who compared the child-rearing practices of the parents of children who were assertive, self-reliant, and self-controlled with the child-rearing practices of the parents of two groups of children who manifested different types of disturbed behavior. Parent dimensions measured were parental control, parental maturity

---

[29] The child-to-environment effect was also observed in a previous study by the author (Kohn, 1966) where the inference was clear that the child was an important determinant of his peers' approach to him.

demands, parental nurturance, and parent-child communication. Her findings were that firmness in disciplinary matters and high expectations of responsible and independent behavior coupled with warmth and clear communication about what was required of the child were associated with competent functioning in 3- to 4-year-old youngsters.

To date, Baumrind's research results on the longitudinal persistence of healthy functioning as related to parental behavior have not been published.

Garmezy as quoted by Pines (1975) has commented on the failure of researchers to study what he called the "invulnerables," children who live in slums, have been exposed to considerable amounts of stress yet flourish in spite of genetic, psychological, or environmental disadvantages. It is likely that a subsample of the group of healthiest children identified in the present investigation would meet Garmezy's criteria of invulnerability.

Garmezy noted that "as much may be learned from studying youngsters who cope exceptionally well as from studying those who break down. In fact, until we do understand the sources of the invulnerable children's strengths, we will be unable to do much effective prevention with the others" (Pines, 1975, p. 7). We would broaden this statement and say that the focus on all youngsters who function with personal strength and competence—whether invulnerable or not—has both theoretical significance for the researcher and practical value for clinicians and mental health specialists who want to modify the course of emotional development and channel it toward relatively adequate social adjustment.

References

Ackerson, L. *Children's behavior problems, I: Incidence, genetic and intellectual factors.* Chicago: University of Chicago Press, 1931.

Ackerson, L. *Children's behavior problems, II: Relative importances and interrelations among traits.* Chicago: University of Chicago Press, 1942.

Anastasi, A. *Differential psychology.* New York: Macmillan, 1958.

Bannister, H., & Ravdin, M. The problem child and his environment. *British Journal of Psychology*, 1944, **34**, part 2.

Barker, R. H., & Wright H. F. *Midwest and its children.* New York: Harper & Row, 1955.

Bateman, B. Learning disorders: A review. *Review of Educational Research*, 1966, **36**, 93–118.

Baumrind, D. Child care practices anteceding three patterns of preschool behavior. *Genetic Psychology Monographs*, 1967, **75**, 43–88.

Baumrind, D., & Black, A. E. Socialization practices associated with dimensions of competence in preschool boys and girls. *Child Development*, 1967, **38**, 291–327.

Bayley, N. Factors influencing the growth of intelligence in young children. *NSSE Yearbook*, 1940, **39**, 49—79.

Bayley, N. Some increasing parent-child similarities during the growth of children. *Journal of Educational Psychology*, 1954, **45**, 1—12.

Bayley, N. Research in child development: A longitudinal perspective. *Merrill-Palmer Quarterly*, 1965, **121**, 183—208.

Bell, R. Q. Convergence: An accelerated longitudinal approach. *Child Development*, 1953, **24**, 142—145.

Bell, R. Q. A reinterpretation of the direction of effects in studies of socialization. *Psychological Review*, 1968, **75**, 81—95.

Bem, D. J., & Allen, A. On predicting some of the people some of the time: The search for cross-situational consistencies in behavior. *Psychological Review*, 1974, **81**, 506—520.

Bennett, I. *Delinquent and neurotic children.* New York: Basic Books, 1960.

Bernstein, B. Social class and linguistic development: A theory of social learning. In A. H. Halsey, J. Flond, & C. A. Anderson (Eds.), *Education, economy and society.* New York: Free Press, 1961.

Biber, B. Integration of mental health principles in the school setting. In G. Caplan (Ed.), *Prevention of mental disorders in children.* New York: Basic Books, 1961.

Biber, B., Gilkeson, E., & Winsor, C. Teacher education at Bank Street College. *The Personnel and Guidance Journal*, 1959, **37**, 559—568.

Biller, H. B. Father absence and the personality development of the child. *Developmental Psychology*, 1970, **2**, 181—201.

Blanchard, R. W. Father availability and academic performance in third grade boys. *Dissertation Abstracts International*, 1970, **30** (11—13), 5232—5233.

Bloom, B. *Stability and change in human characteristics.* New York: Wiley, 1964.

Bonney, M. E. Parents as the makers of social deviates. *Social Forces*, 1941, **20**, 77—87.

Bower, E. M. *Early identification of emotionally handicapped children in school* (2nd ed.). Springfield, Ill.: Thomas, 1969.

Bremer, J. A social psychiatric investigation of a small community in northern Norway. *Acta Psychiatrica et Neurologica*, 1951, Suppl. 62.

Buehler, C. *From birth to maturity.* London: Routledge & Kegan Paul, 1935.

Caldwell, B. M. *Directions for administering and scoring The Preschool Inventory.* Princeton, N.J.: Educational Testing Service, 1967.

Caplan, G. Recent trends in preventive psychiatry. In G. Caplan (Ed.), *Emotional problems of early childhood.* New York: Basic Books, 1955.

Chance, E. *Families in treatment.* New York: Basic Books, 1959.

Clancy, N., & Smither, F. A study of emotionally disturbed children in Santa Barbara County schools. *California Educational Review*, 1953, **4**, 269.

Cohen, J. Multiple regression as a general data-analytic system. *Psychological Bulletin*, 1968, **70**, 426–443.

Cohen, J. *Statistical power analysis for the behavioral sciences.* New York: Academic Press, 1969.

Cohen, J., & Cohen P. *The Quick Test.* New York: Abacus Associates, 1971.

Coleman, J. S. *Equality of educational opportunity.* Washington, D.C.: U.S. Government Printing Office, 1966.

Colligan, J. Personal communication, October 20, 1975.

Conners, C. K. Symptom patterns of hyperkinetic, neurotic, and normal children. *Child Development*, 1970, **41**, 667–682.

Cullen, K. J., & Boundy, C. A. P. Factors relating to behaviour disorders in children. *Australian Paed. Journal*, 1966, **2**, 70–80. (a)

Cullen, K. J., & Boundy, C. A. P. The prevalence of behaviour disorders in the children of 1000 Western Australian families. *Medical Journal of Australia*, 1966, **2**, 805–808. (b)

Cummings, J. D. The incidence of emotional symptoms in school children. *British Journal of Educational Psychology*, 1944, **14**, 151–161.

Danziger, L. Schulreifetests. *Wiener Paed. Ps.*, 1933, **9**.

Dave, R. H. *The identification and measurement of environmental process variables related to intelligence.* Unpublished doctoral dissertation, University of Chicago, 1963.

Davidson, M. Einige untersuchungsergebnisse ueber psychologische stoerungen bei kindern. *Prax. Kinderpsychologie*, 1961, **10**, 273–278.

Davis, A., Gardner, B. B., & Gardner, M. R. The class system of the white caste. In E. E. Maccoby, T. M. Newcomb, & E. L. Hartley (Eds.), *Readings in social psychology* (3rd ed.). New York: Holt, 1958.

Deutsch, M., & Associates. *The disadvantaged child.* New York: Basic Books, 1967.

Deutsch, M., & Brown, B. Social influences in Negro-white intelligence differences. *Journal of Social Issues*, 1964, **20**, 24–25.

Dohrenwend, B. P., & Dohrenwend, B. S. *Social status and psychological disorder.* New York: Wiley, 1969.

Ekstein, R., & Motto, R. L. *From learning for love to love of learning.* New York: Brunner/Mazel, 1969.

Emmerich, W. Structure and development of personal-social behaviors in economically disadvantaged preschool children. *Genetic Psychology Monographs*, 1977 (in press).

Escalona, S., & Leitsch, E. Early phases of personality development: A non-normative study of infant behavior. *Monographs of the Society for Research in Child Development*, 1952, **17** (1, Serial No. 54).

Eysenck, H. J. *The structure of human personality* (3rd ed.). London: Methuen, 1970.

Faris, R. E. L., & Dunham, H. W. *Mental disorders in urban areas: An ecological study of schizophrenia and other psychoses.* Chicago: Chicago University Press, 1939.

Feshbach, S. Aggression. In P. H. Mussen (Ed.), *Carmichael's manual of child psychology*. New York: Wiley, 1970.

Fitzsimmons, M. J. The predictive value of teachers' referrals. In M. Kingman (Ed.), *Orthopsychiatry and the school.* New York: American Orthopsychiatric Association, 1958.

Fleming, P., & Ricks, D. F. Emotions of children before schizophrenia and before character disorder. In M. Roff & D. F. Ricks (Eds.), *Life history research in psychopathology* (Vol. 1). Minneapolis: University of Minnesota Press, 1970.

Freud, A. *Introduction to psycho-analysis for teachers.* London: Allen & Unwin, 1931.

Freud, A. *The psycho-analytical treatment of children.* New York: International Universities Press, 1965. (Originally published, 1946.)

Freud, S. *New introductory lectures on psycho-analysis.* London: Hogarth Press, 1933.

Garmezy, N. Children at risk: The search for the antecedents of schizophrenia. Part I. Conceptual models and research methods. *Schizophrenia Bulletin*, 1974, **8**, 14–90.

Gerth, H. H., & Mills, C. W. (Eds.). *From Max Weber: Essays in sociology.* New York: Oxford University Press, 1946.

Gilbert, G. M. A survey of "referral problems" in metropolitan child guidance centers. *Journal of Clinical Psychology*, 1957, **13**, 37–42.

Golden, M., Birns, B., Bridger, W., & Moss, A. Social class differentiation in cognitive development among black preschool children. *Child Development*, 1971, **42**, 37–45.

Gottesman, I. I. Biogenetics of race and class. In M. Deutsch, I. Katz, & A. R. Jensen (Eds.), *Social class, race and psychological development.* New York: Holt, Rinehart & Winston, 1968.

Gray, S. W., & Klaus, R. A. An experimental preschool program for culturally deprived children. *Child Development*, 1965, **36**, 887–898.

Harman, H. H. *Modern factor analysis.* Chicago: University of Chicago Press, 1967.

Harris, F. D. *Emotional blocks to learning.* Glencoe, Ill.: Free Press, 1961.

Heinicke, C. M., Friedman, D., Prescott, E., Puncel, C., & Sale, J. S. The organization of day care: Considerations relating to the mental health of child and family. *American Journal of Orthopsychiatry*, 1973, **43**, 8–21.

Hewitt, L. E., & Jenkins, R. L. *Fundamental patterns of maladjustment: The dynamics of their origin.* Illinois: D. H. Green, 1946.

Hildreth, J. G., Griffiths, L. N., & McGauvran, N. E. *The Metropolitan Readiness Tests.* New York: Harcourt Brace, 1969.

Himmelweit, H. T. *A factorial study of "children's behavior problems".* Unpublished manuscript, 1952. Cited by Eysenck, H. J. *The structure of human personality* (3rd ed.). London: Methuen, 1970.

Hollingshead, A. B. *Two-factor index of social position.* Unpublished manuscript, 1957. (Available from Department of Sociology, Yale University, New Haven, Conn.)

Hunter, E. C. Changes in teachers' attitude toward children's behavior over the last thirty years. *Mental Hygiene*, 1957, **41**:3.

Irelan, L. M. (Ed.). *Low-income life styles.* Washington, D.C.: U.S. Government Printing Office, 1966.

Jahoda, M. *Current concepts of positive mental health.* New York: Basic Books, 1958.

Jensen, A. R. Social class, race, and genetics: Implications for education. *American Educational Research Journal*, 1968, **5**, 1–42.

Joint Commission on Mental Health of Children. *Crisis in child mental health: Challenge for the 1970's.* New York: Harper & Row, 1969.

Kagan, J., & Moss, H. A. *Birth to maturity: A study in psychological development.* New York: Wiley, 1962.

Kagan, J., Sontag, L. W., Baker, C. T., & Nelson, V. L. Personality and IQ change. *Journal of Abnormal and Social Psychology*, 1958, **56**, 261–266.

Katan, A. Some thoughts about the role of verbalization in early childhood. *The Psychoanalytic Study of the Child.* 1961, **16**, 184–188.

Kessler, J. W. *Psychopathology of childhood.* Englewood Cliffs, N.J.: Prentice-Hall, 1966.

Kohn, M. The child as a determinant of his peers' approach to him. *Journal of Genetic Psychology*, 1966, **109**, 91–100.

Kohn, M. *Competence and symptom factors in the preschool child.* Unpublished manuscript, 1968. (Available from William Alanson White Institute, New York, N.Y. 10023.)

Kohn, M. *The social systems meaning of the two-factor model of social-emotional competence.* Paper presented at the meeting of the American Educational Research Association, Washington, D.C., April 1975.

Kohn, M., & Cohen, J. Emotional impairment and achievement deficit in disadvantaged children—fact or myth? *Genetic Psychology Monographs*, 1975, **92**, 57–78.

Kohn, M., & Rosman, B. L. Therapeutic intervention with disturbed children in day care: Implications of the deprivation hypothesis. *Child Care Quarterly*, 1971, **1**, 21–46.

Kohn, M., & Rosman, B. L. Relationship of preschool social-emotional functioning to later intellectual achievement. *Developmental Psychology*, 1972, **6**, 445–452. (a)

Kohn, M., & Rosman, B. L. A Social Competence Scale and Symptom Checklist for the preschool child: Factor dimensions, their cross-instrument generality, and longitudinal persistence. *Developmental Psychology*, 1972, **6**, 430–444. (b)

Kohn, M., & Rosman, B. L. Cognitive functioning in five-year-old boys as related to social-emotional and background variables. *Developmental Psychology*, 1973, **8**, 277–294. (a)

Kohn, M., & Rosman, B. L. Cross-situational and longitudinal stability of social-emotional functioning in young children. *Child Development*, 1973, **44**, 721–727. (b)

Kohn, M., & Rosman, B. L. A two-factor model of emotional disturbance in the young child: Validity and screening efficiency. *Journal of Child Psychology and Psychiatry*, 1973, **14**, 31–56. (c)

Kohn, M., & Rosman, B. L. Social-emotional, cognitive and demographic determinants of poor school achievement: Implications for a strategy of intervention. *Journal of Educational Psychology*, 1974, **66**, 267–276.

Koretzky, M. *An examination of human consistency and background-risk through the Two-Factor Model of Social-Emotional Functioning.* Unpublished doctoral dissertation, State University of New York at Stony Brook, 1976.

Koretzky, M., & Kohn, M. *Cross-situational consistency among problem adolescents: An application of the two-factor model.* Unpublished manuscript, 1976. (Available from Jewish Board of Guardians, New York, N.Y. 10019.)

Langner, T. S., Goff, J. A., Greene, E. L., Herson, J. H., & Jameson, J. D. Children of the city: Affluence, poverty and mental health. In V. L. Allen (Ed.), *Psychological factors in poverty.* Chicago: Markham, 1970.

Langner, T. S., Goff, J. A., Greene, E. L., Herson, J. H., Jameson, J. D., & McCarthy, E. *Psychiatric impairment in welfare and nonwelfare city children.* Paper presented at the meeting of the American Psychological Association, Washington, D. C., September 1969.

Lapouse, R., & Monk, M. A. An epidemiologic study of behavior characteristics in children. *American Journal of Public Health*, 1958, **48**, 1134–1144.

Lapouse, R., & Monk, M. A. Behavior deviations in a representative sample of children: Variation by sex, age, race, social class, and family size. *American Journal of Orthopsychiatry*, 1964, **34**, 436—446.

Laycock, S. R. Teachers' reactions to maladjustment of school children. *British Journal of Educational Psychology*, 1934, **4**:11.

Levy, D. M. *Maternal over-protection.* New York: Columbia University Press, 1943.

Lewis, H. *Deprived children.* London: Oxford University Press, 1954.

Lindeman, E. Symptomatology and management of acute grief. *American Journal of Psychiatry*, 1944, **101**, 141—148.

Lindeman, E. B., & Ross, A. A follow-up study of a predictive test of social adaptation in preschool children. In G. Caplan (Ed.), *Emotional problems of early childhood.* New York: Basic Books, 1955.

Lorr, M., Klett, C. J., & McNair, D. M. *Syndromes of psychosis.* New York: Pergamon Press, 1963.

Lurie, O. R. The emotional health of children in the family setting. *Community Mental Health Journal*, 1970, **6**, 229—235.

Macfarlane, J. W., Allen, L., & Honzik, M. P. *A developmental study of the behavior problems of normal children between twenty-one months and fourteen years.* Berkeley, Calif.: University of California Press, 1954.

Maes, W. R. The identification of emotionally disturbed elementary school children. *Exceptional Child*, 1966, **33**:607.

McClelland, D. C. *The achieving society.* Princeton, N.J.: Van Nostrand, 1961.

McCord, J., McCord, W., & Thurber, E. Some effect of paternal absence on male children. *Journal of Abnormal and Social Psychology*, 1962, **64**, 361—369.

McFie, B. S. Behaviour and personality difficulties in school children. *British Journal of Educational Psychology*, 1934, **4**:30.

McNemar, Q. *Psychological statistics.* New York: Wiley, 1969.

Mensh, I. N., Kantor, M. B., Domke, H. R., Gildea, M. C. L., & Glidewell, J. C. Children's behavior symptoms and their relationship to school adjustment, sex, and social class. *Journal of Social Issues*, 1959, **15**, 8—15.

Michael, L. M., Morris, D. P., & Soroker, E. Follow-up studies of shy, withdrawn children II: Relative incidence of schizophrenia. *American Journal of Orthopsychiatry*, 1957, **27**, 331—337.

Michael, S. T. Psychiatrist's commentary. In Srole, L., Langner, T. S., Michael, S. T., Opler, M. K., & Rennie, T. A. C. *Mental health in the metropolis.* New York: McGraw-Hill, 1962.

Minuchin, P., Biber, B., Shapiro, E., & Zimiles, H. *The psychological impact of the school experience.* New York: Basic Books, 1969.

Mischel, W. *Personality and assessment.* New York: Wiley, 1968.

Mitchell, B. C. Personal communication, May 14, 1975.

Mitchell, J. A. A study of teachers' and mental hygienists' ratings of certain behavior problems of children. *Journal of Educational Review*, 1942, **36**:292.

Mitchell, S. *A study of mental health of school children in an English county.* Unpublished doctoral dissertation, University of London, 1965.

Moles, O. C., Jr. Training children in low-income families for school. *Welfare in Review*, 1965, **3**(6), 1–11.

Morris, D. P., Soroker, E., & Burruss, G. Follow-up studies of shy, withdrawn children—I: Evaluation of later adjustment. *American Journal of Orthopsychiatry*, 1954, **24**, 743–754.

Morris, H. H., Escoll, P. J., & Wexler, R. Aggressive behavior disorders in childhood—A follow-up study. *American Journal of Psychiatry*, 1956, **112**, 991–997.

Mulligan, D. G. *Some correlates of maladjustment in a national sample of school children.* Unpublished doctoral dissertation, University of London, 1964.

Murray, H. A. *Explorations in personality.* New York: Oxford University Press, 1938.

Nameche, G., Waring, M., & Ricks, D. Early indicators of outcome in schizophrenia. *Journal of Nervous and Mental Disease,* 1964, **139**, 232–240.

Nye, F. I. *Family relationships and delinquent behavior.* New York: Wiley, 1958.

Olson, W. C. *Problem tendencies in children.* Minneapolis: University of Minnesota Press, 1930.

Orpet, R. E., & Meyers, C. E. Factorially established rubrics of observations of test behavior. *Journal of Clinical Psychology*, 1963, **19**, 292–294.

Pasamanick, B., & Knobloch, H. Epidemiologic studies on the complications of pregnancy and the birth process. In G. Caplan (Ed.), *Prevention of mental disorders in children.* New York: Basic Books, 1961.

Patterson, G. R. An empirical approach to the classification of disturbed children. *Journal of Clinical Psychology*, 1964, **20**, 326–337.

Pauly, F. R. Let's give boys a break. *Phi Delta Kappan*, 1959 (April), 281–283.

Paynter, R. H., & Blanchard, P. *A study of educational achievement of problem children.* New York: Commonwealth Fund, 1929.

Pearson, J. H. A survey of learning difficulties in children. *The Psychoanalytic Study of the Child*, 1952, **7**, 322–386.

Peterson, D. R. The age generality of personality factors derived from ratings. *Educational and Psychological Measurement*, 1960, **20**, 461–474.

Peterson, D. R. Behavior problems of middle childhood. *Journal of Consulting Psychology*, 1961, **25**, 205–209.

Peterson, D. R. Scope and generality of verbally defined personality factors. *Psychological Review*, 1965, **72**, 48–57.

Peterson, D. R. *A clinical study of social behavior.* New York: Appleton-Century-Crofts, 1968.

Peterson, D. R., Becker, W. C., Shoemaker, D. J., Luria, Z., & Hellmer, L. A. Child behavior problems and parental attitudes. *Child Development*, 1961, **32**, 355–372.

Peterson, D. R., Quay, H. C., & Cameron, J. R. Personality and background factors in juvenile delinquency as inferred from questionnaire responses. *Journal of Consulting Psychology*, 1959, **23**, 395–399.

Pines, M. Infants are smarter than anybody thinks. *New York Times Magazine*, November 29, 1970.

Pines, M. In praise of "invulnerables". *APA Monitor*, December 1975, p. 7.

Prescott, E., & Jones, E. *Group day care as a child-rearing environment.* Unpublished manuscript, Pacific Oaks College, 1967.

President's Commission on Law Enforcement and Administration of Justice. *Task force report: Juvenile delinquency and youth crime.* Washington, D.C.: U.S. Government Printing Office, 1967.

Pringle, M. L. K., Butler, N., & Davie, R. *11,000 seven-year-olds.* New York: Humanities Press, 1966.

Raven, J. C. *Colored progressive matrices.* London: Harrap, 1956.

Richards, H. C., & McCandless, B. R. Socialization dimensions among five-year-old slum children. *Journal of Educational Psychology*, 1972, **63**, 44–55.

Ricks, D. F., & Berry, J. C. Family and symptom patterns that precede schizophrenia. In M. Roff & D. F. Ricks (Eds.), *Life history research in psychopathology* (Vol. 1). Minneapolis: University of Minnesota Press, 1970.

Ricks, D. F., & Nameche, G. F. Symbiosis, sacrifice and schizophrenia. *Mental Hygiene*, 1966, **50**, 11–15.

Risley, T. R., & Baer, D. M. Operant behavior modification: The deliberate development of behavior. In B. M. Caldwell & H. N. Ricciuti (Eds.), *Review of child development research* (Vol. 3). Chicago: University of Chicago Press, 1973.

Robins, L. N. *Deviant children grown up.* Baltimore, Md.: Williams & Wilkins, 1966.

Roff, M. A. A factorial study of the Fels Parent Behavior Scales. *Child Development*, 1949, **20**, 29–45.

Rogers, C. A. Mental health findings in the elementary school. *Educational Review Bulletin*, Ohio State University, 1942, **21**:3.

Ross, A. O., Lacy, H. M., & Parton, D. A. The development of a behavior checklist for boys. *Child Development*, 1965, **36**, 1013–1027.

Rutter, M. Classification and categorization in child psychiatry. *International Journal of Psychiatry*, 1967, **3**, 161–167.

Rutter, M., Tizard, J., & Whitmore, K. *Education, health and behavior.* New York: Wiley, 1970.

Ryle, A., Pond, D. A., & Hamilton, M. The prevalence and patterns of psychological disturbance in children of primary age. *Journal of Child Psychology and Psychiatry*, 1965, **6**, 101–113.

Sameroff, A. J., & Chandler, M. J. Reproductive risk and the continuum of caretaking casualty. In F. D. Horowitz (Ed.), *Review of child development research* (Vol. 4). Chicago: University of Chicago Press, 1975.

Sanford, R. N., Adkins, M. M., Miller, R. B., & Cobb, E. A. Physique, personality and scholarship. *Monographs of the Society for Research in Child Development*, 1943, **7** (Serial No. 34).

Schaefer, E. S. Converging conceptual models for maternal behavior and for child behavior. In J. C. Glidewell (Ed.), *Parental attitudes and child behavior.* Springfield, Ill.: Thomas, 1961.

Schaefer, E. S. Development of hierarchical, configurational models for parent and child behavior. In J. P. Hill (Ed.), *Minnesota symposium on child psychology* (Vol. 5). Minneapolis: University of Minnesota Press, 1971.

Schaefer, E. S. *Major replicated dimensions of adjustment and achievement: Cross-cultural, cross-sectional, and longitudinal research.* Paper presented at the meeting of the American Educational Research Association, Washington, D.C., April 1975.

Schaefer, E. S., & Aaronson, M. R. *Classroom Behavior Inventory: Preschool to primary.* Unpublished manuscript, 1966. (Available from School of Public Health, University of North Carolina, Chapel Hill, N.C.)

Schaefer, E. S., Droppleman, L. F., & Kalverboer, A. F. *Development of a classroom behavior check list and factor analyses of children's school behavior in the United States and the Netherlands.* Unpublished manuscript, 1965. (Available from School of Public Health, University of North Carolina, Chapel Hill, N.C.)

Schrupp, M. H., & Gjerde, C. M. Teacher growth in attitudes toward behavior problems of children. *Journal of Educational Psychology*, 1953, **44**, 203–214.

Sexton, P. C. *Education and income.* New York: Viking Press, 1961.

Shepherd, M., Oppenheim, B., & Mitchell, S. *Childhood behavior and mental health.* New York: Grune & Stratton, 1971.

Sontag, L. W., Baker, C. T., & Nelson, V. L. Mental growth and personality development: A longitudinal study. *Monographs of the Society for Research in Child Development*, 1958, **23** (2, Serial No. 67).

Srole, L., Langner, T. S., Michael, S. T., Opler, M. K., & Rennie, T. A. C. *Mental health in the metropolis*. New York: McGraw-Hill, 1962.

Stabenau, J. R., & Pollin, W. Experiential differences for schizophrenics as compared with their non-schizophrenic siblings: Twin and family studies. In M. Roff & D. F. Ricks (Eds.), *Life history research in psychopathology*. Minneapolis: University of Minnesota Press, 1970.

Stennett, R. J. Emotional handicaps in the elementary school years: Phase or disease? *American Journal of Orthopsychiatry*, 1966, **36**, 444–449.

Stern, G. G. *People in context*. New York: Wiley, 1970.

Stott, D. H. A new delinquency prediction instrument using behavioural indications. *International Journal of Social Psychiatry*, 1960, **6**, 195–205.

Symonds, P. M. *The psychology of parent-child relationships*. New York: Appleton-Century-Crofts, 1939.

Tyler, L. E. *The psychology of human differences*. New York: Appleton-Century-Crofts, 1965.

Ullman, C. A. *Identification of maladjusted school children* (Public Health Monograph #7). Washington, D.C.: U.S. Government Printing Office, 1952.

von Harnack, G. A. *Wesen und soziale bedingtheit fruehkindlicher verhaltensstoerungen*. Basel: S. Karger, 1953.

Waring, M., & Ricks, D. F. Family patterns of children who become adult schizophrenics. *Journal of Nervous and Mental Disease*, 1965, **140**, 351–364.

Wasserman, H. L. Father-absent and father-present lower-class Negro families: A comparative study of family functioning. *Dissertation Abstracts*, 1969, **29**, 4569–4570.

Watt, N. F. Longitudinal changes in the social behavior of children hospitalized for schizophrenia as adults. *Journal of Nervous and Mental Disease*, 1972, **155**, 42–54.

Watt, N. F. Childhood and adolescent routes to schizophrenia. In D. F. Ricks, A. Thomas, & M. Roff (Eds.), *Life history research in psychopathology* (Vol. 3). Minneapolis: University of Minnesota Press, 1974.

Watt, N. F., Stolorow, R. D., Lubensky, A. W., & McClelland, D. C. School adjustment and behavior of children hospitalized for schizophrenia as adults. *American Journal of Orthopsychiatry*, 1970, **40**, 637–657.

Wenar, C., & Wenar, S. C. The short term prospective model, the illusion of time, and the tabula rasa child. *Child Development*, 1963, **34**, 697–708.

White, R. W. *Lives in progress.* New York: Dryden Press, 1952.

Whiteman, M., & Deutsch, M. Social disadvantage as related to intellective and language development. In M. Deutsch, I. Katz, & A. R. Jensen (Eds.), *Social class, race and psychological development.* New York: Holt, Rinehart & Winston, 1968.

Wickman, E. K. *Children's behavior and teacher's attitudes.* New York: Commonwealth Fund, 1928.

Wolf, R. M. *The identification and measurement of environmental process variables related to intelligence.* Unpublished doctoral dissertation, University of Chicago, 1963.

Wynne, L. C. *Children and families vulnerable to schizophrenia.* Unpublished manuscript, 1972. (Available from Department of Psychiatry, University of Rochester School of Medicine, Rochester, N.Y.)

Author Index

A

Aaronson, M. R., 18, 36, 37, 50, 69
Ackerson, L., 14, 15, 17, 36, 100, 250
Adkins, M. M., 261
Allen, A., 252
Allen, L., 6
Anastasi, A., 119, 120

B

Baer, D. M., 251
Baker, C. T., 231
Bannister, H., 24
Barker, R. H., 251
Bateman, B., 8
Baumrind, D., 266, 267
Bayley, N., 207, 232
Becker, W. C., 251
Bell, R. Q., 259, 260, 266
Bem, D. J., 252
Bennett, I., 20, 175
Bernstein, B., 6, 232
Berry, J. C., 31, 33, 252, 264
Biber, B., 102, 118
Biller, H. B., 141, 175
Birns, B., 232
Black, A. E., 266
Blanchard, P., 14, 16
Blanchard, R. W., 207
Bloom, B., 63
Bonney, M. E., 24

Boundy, C. A. P., 98, 101, 175
Bower, E. M., 8, 58, 60, 98, 117, 175, 202, 206
Bremer, J., 99
Bridger, W., 232
Brown, B., 207
Buehler, C., 62
Burruss, G., 25
Butler, N., 120, 175

C

Caldwell, B. M., 203
Cameron, J. R., 20
Caplan, G., 102, 241
Chance, E., 41, 42
Chandler, M. J., 258, 266
Clancy, N., 4
Cobb, E. A., 262
Cohen, J., 63, 89, 137, 138, 208
Cohen, P., 89
Coleman, J. S., 4, 126, 208, 232
Colligan, J., 128
Conners, C. K., 20
Cullen, K. J., 98, 101, 175
Cummings, J. D., 24, 98, 100, 101

D

Danziger, L., 62

Subject Index[1]

A

Academic attainment measures, of present study

See Academic Standing, Arithmetic Achievement, Grade Placement, Level Within Grade, Metropolitan Readiness Test, Verbal Achievement, Verbal Fluency

Academic Standing, 73, 205

definition of, 64

findings of present study, 121, 123-124, 126, 223-224, 226-227

Acting-out behavior

See Anger-Defiance, Low Task Orientation

Age 57, 140, 141, 146, 149, 155, 158, 206, 207, 210, 216

and symptom changes, 100-101

trends in academic attainment, 122-129

trends in healthy functioning, 183-188, 191-192, 193-194

trends in level of disturbance, 105-114, 117-118, 127-129, 162-168, 176-177, 183-191, 192-193

Anger-Defiance 2, 20, 53, 58, 60

as outcome measure, 139, 148-152, 153, 157-162

as predictor of emotional impairment

findings of present study, 146-147, 149-150, 152, 155, 156, 158-160, 162

hypotheses, 143, 153, 154

as predictor of underachievement

findings of present study, 210-212, 214-219, 223-230, 247-249

hypotheses, 208

definition of, 43-46, 236

reliability of, 46, 66-68

stability of cross-syndrome longitudinal correlations, 170-171, 172-174, 196-197

stability of same-syndrome longitudinal correlations, 170-172, 173-174

validity of, 81-96, 114-116, 139, 147, 156, 178, 238

See also Age trends in level of disturbance, Circumplex model of social-emotional functioning, Cooperation-Compliance, Sex differences in emotional impairment

Apathy-Withdrawal, 2, 20, 53, 58, 60

as outcome measure, 139, 148-152, 153, 157-162

as predictor of emotional impairment

findings of present study, 146-147,

---

[1] Subjects in *italics* refer to the variables of the longitudinal study.